PRAISE FOR *MAKE PEACE WITH YOUR PLATE*

"Jess Ainscough is a wellness warrior of the finest kind. Her journey will deeply inspire you to transform your life."

– Kris Carr, *New York Times* best selling author, *Crazy Sexy Kitchen*

"Inspiring, practical, funny & heart wrenching. A no-nonsense guide to eating clean and feeling great. *Make Peace With Your Plate* makes eating healthy fun! Cancer Thriver turned Wellness Warrior Jess Aisncough takes you on her miraculous journey with food. You'll discover her secrets to eating like a clean queen."

– James Colquhoun, International Best-Selling Filmmaker Food Matters & Hungry For Change

"Jess is a leading force in the new way of thinking about health and wellness. *Make Peace With Your Plate* will not only inspire you, but it will give you the tools you truly need to make sustainable changes to your life."

– Dr Frank Lipman

MAKE PEACE WITH
YOUR PLATE

Make Peace With Your Plate

Change Your Life
One Meal at a Time

JESS AINSCOUGH

HAY HOUSE, INC.
Carlsbad, California • New York City
London • Sydney • Johannesburg
Vancouver • Hong Kong • New Delhi

To my incredible support team –
Mum, Dad, Tallon and Edie.
You guys are always
right at the top of my gratitude list.

CONTENTS

FOREWORD

ᨒ Several years ago, the front cover of one of the local Sunshine Coast magazines showed a picture of a beautiful young girl with long blond hair wearing a dress made from cabbage leaves. That got me curious. I'm a nutritionist and anything about food makes me sit up and pay attention.

I flipped through the magazine until I got to the article of the girl in the cabbage leaf dress. Her story was hard to pull myself away from and, at the end of the article, I noticed that she didn't live far from me. I found a way to contact her and let her know that she was a shining light for young people's health.

It's important to let people know—those who are going against the conventional wisdom of medicine today—that they are on the right track and that what they are doing will not only help their own health but those of people who follow their lead.

Jessica Ainscough was the girl in the cabbage leaf dress. Her story was and is compelling, and her quest to cure her cancer unconventionally and alone was and has been heroic.

Health is something many people don't have, or that they take for granted. They have been brought up in a generation where processed and modified foods are normal, while eating foods from nature only happens on occasion. Disease rates are rising to catastrophic levels: many children have the health of the elderly and many of the elderly are spending decades debilitated with sickness. They don't know what it is to feel good and, if they don't have a current health crisis, they continue to abuse their bodies with alcohol, drugs and poor food choices until a health crisis hits them and flattens their energy and vitality.

This is what happened to Jessica. She had the biggest wake-up call of her life and at a very young age. Hindsight is a wonderful thing and, after it happens, we wish we'd had the foresight. This is how I felt the first time I had dinner with Jessica Ainscough. Let me explain.

My belief is that the body is continually letting you know if something is wrong. At first it whispers: small headaches, aches, pains, a continuous runny nose, tiredness, stopped periods, sore hands and small niggling things that you can take a pill for to make the symptoms go away. If you don't deal with the whispers, the body begins to scream at you with continuous migraines, arthritic changes, constant colds and flu, chronic fatigue, infertility, diabetes, cancer and heart disease.

I asked Jessica if she had had any warning signs early in her life regarding her health. I wanted to know if her body had been whispering to her that something was wrong. Jessica told me that she knew things were not right with her health in her teenage years but, like most people, she ignored the whispers. However she found she couldn't ignore the screams of cancer.

This is what happens to many people. They ignore the whispers until one day they can't keep going and are stopped in their tracks. I see this as an opportunity for change. After all, they are where they are because of the choices they have made. So, in order to get out of where they are, they have to make different choices. Most people just continue on with their lives, making no lifestyle changes and giving the responsibility for their health to someone else, with potions and medicines that may or may not cure them.

It takes strength, persistence and courage to make permanent change in life; it all depends on how desperate you become. It also takes strength to not just follow the crowd.

I don't believe there are any mistakes. I believe Jessica Ainscough's path in life was to experience the big C; and not just any old cancer but epithelioid sarcoma and at a very young age. Her journey to discovering what health is and how to achieve it has been monumental. And with her knowledge and awakening, she has hauled with her a plethora of people who love to read her daily blogs on her awakening. I was one of them.

Jessica is a shining light, a beacon who writes in such a compelling and honest way that she reaches those who perhaps would not be reached. This book, *Make Peace With Your Plate,* tells the raw and scary truth of a young girl who didn't listen to her body and paid the price. Her story will draw you in and lead you to the steps you need to follow, in order to find foods and tools that heal. Jessica's experience and knowledge will guide you.

Whether you are in a crisis or are looking for information on how to find and maintain health, this book has the information you need to set you on a journey that will profoundly alter your health—both physically and mentally.

I am so honoured to count Jessica as one of my friends and colleagues. Her fate, her destiny, is to be an educator of health and this book is just the beginning. Read and take action, as knowledge is powerful. And acting on that knowledge will give the solutions you are seeking for longevity, health, energy and vitality.

Happy changing habits.

Cyndi O'Meara

Nutritionist, author, speaker and founder of *Changing Habits*

INTRODUCTION

∞∞∞ You have no idea how long I've been waiting for this day. Ever since I made my debut into the world of wellness (you know, when I walked out and curtsied in a gown made of cabbage leaves and a bouquet of broccoli!) I've been waiting for the moment when I would have a platform large enough to match the size and importance of the message I yearned to pass on. This day has come; and the aforementioned platform is the glorious book your eyes are dancing over right now. And so it's time to impart the message. Brace yourself, because it's a game changer. Here goes …

Being healthy, losing weight, looking amazing and feeling phenomenal does not mean that you have to surrender to a lifetime of deprivation, dieting, counting calories and eating boring and bland food.

Being healthy, losing weight, looking amazing and feeling phenomenal does not mean that you have to give up the foods your taste buds go wild over.

Being healthy, losing weight, looking amazing and feeling phenomenal does not mean that you need to torture yourself every time you look at a piece of chocolate cake, and then become ravaged with guilt every time you break a promise to yourself by eating it.

No, no, no! That kind of thinking is old school. It's outdated. It's going to go and live with reruns of the original *Beverly Hills 90210*.

Consider this scenario instead:

> *What would your life look like if you could eat whatever you wanted, and yet look in the mirror and see someone you were completely in love with staring back at you?*
>
> *Imagine how much space you would have in your mind if it weren't occupied by so many destructive thoughts about food and, more importantly, what your food choices are doing to your ass, thighs, stomach or whatever other area of your body you pinch and look at in disgust. Imagine how much energy you would have, how much happier you would be and how much more you would get done, if worrying about your weight and food choices just didn't exist.*

Most of us have such a tortured relationship with our food that we are forever caught up in a vicious cycle of deprivation, indulgence and guilt. What if I were to tell you that deprivation and guilt don't need a place in this dysfunctional threesome? What if I were to tell you that there is a 'whole' way of eating, where the food you love is also the food that your body, mind and the planet loves? This means that you would never have to worry about your weight again!

Think I'm yanking your chain? I'm not. You see, some-where along the line, the way we perceive food has got incredibly messed up. Have you ever thought about why we were given taste buds? It wasn't so that God (or Goddess, Buddha, the Universe, Source, Baby Jesus—whomever you believe is up there) could sit on his or her cloud and torture us every time we try to satisfy our taste buds with a packet of chips or a chocolate muffin. No, we were given a taste for sweet treats and salty flavours for a reason. It's just that with all of the packaged, processed and chemicalised 'food-like substances' that line the aisles of our supermarkets, most of us have no idea how to silence cravings without adding an extra inch to that muffin top. It doesn't have to be like this. There is another way.

I know I've mentioned 'weight' several times already, but the message I want to express isn't really about being skinny. Achieving your ideal weight is a major part of it, but only because it's a superficial side effect of getting your insides in tiptop shape. My message is about wellness: whole body, complete, total, feel-so-good-you-feel-like-you're-leaving-a-trail-of-rainbow-sparkles-wherever-you-go wellness. It's about learning what foods deserve to be in your beautiful body and which ones don't even deserve to be called food.

I'm going to take you on a journey back to a time when things were simpler. When food consisted of Mother Nature's magic, rather than the numbered gibberish we read on the back of ingredients labels. A time when we didn't need a science textbook to decipher nutrition claims and when foods had a shelf life shorter than our attention span. A time when we weren't tempted by quick fix plans and powdered detox promises that would have our ancestors considering us completely crazy. And then, we're going to discuss easy ways to implement these principles into modern day life.

I know you're busy and I know that, when you're feeling stretched for time, the last thing you consider doing is dropping everything to don an apron and whip up a nutritious meal from scratch. But that doesn't mean it's time to scrap all considerations of health and wellness and eat microwaved dinners. I shudder at the thought. And by the time you've finished reading this book, you will too.

Eating should be about enjoyment. It should be about feeding your body the best quality foods, so that you can live a long, healthy and authentic life—so that you can be the best version of you. The food we eat forms the basis of our lives. It determines whether we are healthy, happy and showing up each day in a way that is in alignment with our greatest hopes and dreams. It's criminal to rob yourself of this opportunity.

This book is not about overwhelming you with more confusing and contradicting rules. The fight isn't about whether we eat meat or not, or whether we follow a raw diet, a vegan diet or a Paleo diet. In my opinion, the battle ends when we stop shovelling chemicalised crap into our bodies and start feeding ourselves with real food.

I'm not into diets, but if I had to give this one a name it would be the *Real Food Diet*. Or, the *Common Sense Diet*. Or, the *Eat-What-Your-Body-Runs-Best-On Diet*. This is also where peace can be cultivated. On top of everything else, we don't need to feel bad about the fact that we aren't vegan, or we like cooked food every now and then, or we can't quite get the idea of eating like Paleo. This book is not about that. It's about accepting that we're not all the same. We all work differently, fuelled by different foods.

What I'm striving to share is the simple beauty of creating a culinary foundation based on the natural laws of the earth: eat food that Mother Nature provides and you can't go wrong. Whatever comes after that is a personal decision, and it's one that no-one else can make but you. Read the information I'm about to share with you, go away and research other dietary theories, experiment with different foods and food preparation styles, and then come to a conclusion about what works best for you. That is the basis of empowerment. That is the best and simplest way to do away with the torture of dieting, and to be at complete peace with the food on your plate.

We're not just going to deal with the food you eat though. Making peace with your plate involves so much more than paying attention to the grub you put in your gob.

In the third part of this book, we're going to venture beyond our plates and take a look at all of the other areas of your life that contribute to your overall health and well-ness—which is pretty much everything. In the spirit of not turning this into a never-ending story, I'm just going to go into the main ones: self-love, relationships, sunlight, movement, living on purpose and spirituality. We'll also dive deep into the mindset behind creating a permanent, healthy lifestyle transformation; so that everything you learn and start putting into practice becomes a natural part of your life that you never even consider straying from. Not because you're afraid to, but because you feel too damn good to ever want to settle for mediocre again!

One more thing before we get started. This book is best read with an open mind. Some of the information you read may ruffle your feathers and meet with a bit of resistance. This is a completely normal reaction when we hear something that challenges what has always been accepted as truth. One of our daily challenges is to keep an open, beginner's mind when we're faced with information that takes us off guard. When that happens, keep this quote in mind:

> *All truth passes through three stages. First, it is ridiculed. Second, it is violently opposed. Third, it is accepted as being self-evident.*
>
> ∞ Arthur Schopenhauer

Right on, Arthur.

I hope that this book brings you the incredibly freeing food liberation intended. I hope that, after you've read these pages and allowed my words to soak in, you'll hold food up on the pedestal that it deserves. The aim of the game is for you to have a mutually-beneficial relationship with your food: that you love your food and that it loves you right back.

WELLNESS WARRIOR

PART ONE

THE WELLNESS WARRIOR STORY

∞ Let's travel back in time for a moment, to when I was 15 years old. If you asked 15-year-old me what she wanted to be when she grew up, the last thing she would have said is a wellness advocate. I wanted to be a journalist ever since I was a wee lass (I won a bike helmet in an essay writing competition when I was 10 and decided that was a gift I should leverage), and there were brief periods when I thought a career as a hairdresser or a fashion designer sounded like fun. But health? Nothing sounded more boring than a whole career revolving around watching what you eat. I come from a family of enthusiastic eaters—I can't stand having to share my food with anyone, and I always won eating competitions when faced with an all-you-can-eat buffet.

My almost insatiable appetite—which I would try to satiate with meat pies, chicken burgers, hot chips, chocolate chip muffins and other such junk—didn't start working against me until my mid teens. Suddenly, I went from thin and athletic to chunky … with cellulite. This physical transition was also accompanied by a psychological shift. I began hating myself and my body, no longer immune to the onslaught of the toxic foods I was feeding it.

It was also around this time that I started bolstering my lifestyle with drugs and booze. I smoked weed for the first time in my early teens and a year or so later I was drinking until I puked almost every weekend. I was arrested at the end of Grade 10 for underage drinking and being drunk and disorderly in a public place. My parents had to pick me up from the back of a police car (they'd been at a fancy dress party and were wearing makeshift togas made from bed sheets). When I was 16, all of the binge drinking had destroyed my liver to the point where a doctor warned me that, if I kept it up, I would end up with premature cirrhosis of the liver—a condition usually affecting middle-aged alcoholics, not teenage girls. Once I turned 18, I spent every weekend in a nightclub, and I initiated a tumultuous relationship with party drugs. I fell in love with ecstasy the first time I tried it (the book *Anna's Story* did absolutely nothing to deter me) and pretty soon I was so dependent on pills that I didn't think I could have a fun night out without them. I was having an absolute ball … until about 6am every Sunday, when the come down pity party made me depressed and self-loathing.

As soon as I graduated from university, I moved to Sydney to start my career as a magazine writer. My first job involved reporting on the Sydney social scene. I felt like the luckiest girl alive. I'd moved from the Sunshine Coast, a relatively small town, to an exciting big city and it was my 'job' to go out every night to glamorous parties! I had no idea how to cook when I left home, so my diet consisted of canapés at parties and late-night microwave meals (and a steady stream of champagne and cocktails). I went to work with a hangover most mornings, but it was never so bad that a greasy bacon and egg roll couldn't fix it. Unless you count that morning when I threw up in the car on the way to work. I was all class.

Along with the canapés and cocktails, cocaine also made a grand entrance into my life. I could never afford to buy it on my measly salary, but it was on offer at many of the parties I attended. In hindsight, one would consider snorting cocaine off toilet seats at clubs a low point, but at the time I was having an absolute blast.

My second job in Sydney was as the online editor for *Dolly* magazine, a teen girl's bible. This was the dream job for a girl in her early 20s (ironically reporting on issues like the dangers of binge drinking and party drugs). Everything was working according to plan. I had an awesome job, a boyfriend who gave me the freedom to run as wild as I pleased, and an awesome group of friends to share it all with. I was leading a lifestyle that was definitely not very good for me, but it was so much fun that I would never have given any of it up without something drastic happening first. Which it did, but we will get to that in a jiffy.

Back then, my relationship with food was anything but peaceful. I thought that food was something to be enjoyed while it was in my mouth, and then loathed when I looked in the mirror. I've never been overweight, but I constantly hated my body. I had big thighs, a big ass, wobbly arms and my face was just so round. This is what I told myself, anyway. I thought that healthy eating consisted of choosing the low-fat version of my favourite foods, then avoiding anything that tasted good if my jeans started getting too tight. I couldn't cook. If my boyfriend didn't cook for me, I would eat packet pasta, packet rice, microwave pies or just call up my friends at the Thai restaurant. All of this was complemented by guilt and empty promises of working it all off at the gym. I worked long hours and told myself that I didn't have time to experiment with anything in the kitchen.

Back then, I didn't know any better. I honestly didn't think there was anything wrong with my diet or the way I was living. I was young and I was healthy. Or so I thought. It wasn't until my life was stamped with a looming expiry date that I was forced to take a glaring look at the really detrimental effects of my lifestyle.

At 9am on 24 April 2007, I slipped away from my desk at *Dolly* magazine and walked excitedly to my hand doctor's office. Two weeks prior I'd had surgery to remove fluid on my left middle finger and biopsies to work out why I had strange little lumps popping up all over my hand and arm. The cast I'd had to wear for the two weeks was a drag. It was uncomfortable and impossible to hide in photographs, and I felt peeved about having to type with one hand at work. With the MTV awards just two days away, I was keen to get the thing off.

'We've got the results of your biopsies' my doctor said, straight after he'd removed the bulky cast and replaced it with a smaller bandage '... and it's not good news I'm afraid.' I was confused. What the heck was he talking about? I stared at him with a blank look as he continued. 'The results have told us that you have a rare type of cancer called epithelioid sarcoma.' I went numb. 'It's not treatable with chemotherapy or radiation and there's a good chance we will have to amputate your arm. But this disease is essentially terminal.'

This was the sentence that summoned a dark cloud into the room and sent chills down my spine. In the space of about 20 minutes, I'd gone from being a happy, enthusiastic magazine writer, living the life I'd dreamt of for so long, to ... a terminal cancer patient? I was just 22 years old and had just been told that I had hundreds of tumours in my left hand, arm and up into my armpit. I was also told that there was basically nothing that could be done to save me and that the only way to give me some extra time on this planet was to chop my whole arm off.

With no knowledge whatsoever about cancer, apart from the fact that Kylie Minogue had survived it, I was eager to do whatever my doctors told me to do—everything except have my arm amputated. That just didn't seem right to me. It may very well have been vanity speaking, but something told me that cutting my arm off was wrong. However, I felt that by refusing to do what they were telling me, I would let my family down. Seeing the pain my diagnosis caused them broke my heart. Sitting there while the doctor told them that, without an amputation, I would be dead within a few years was too much. So, I signed the papers and booked in to have my arm cut off then sunk into a dark depression. Everything felt so wrong.

Someone else must have thought so too because, three days before I was scheduled to have the operation, I received a call from my doctor offering me another solution. He wanted to try out an isolated limb infusion and pump an extremely high dose of chemotherapy through my arm. I was told that it was 10 times as potent as what they put into the body (my arm was tied off with a tourniquet to prevent the chemo entering the rest of my body). I was told that if the same amount of chemo had entered my body, I would have been dead in an instant.

With my only other option being amputation, I eagerly agreed to the limb infusion. I spent nine days in hospital having and recovering from the procedure, nursing an intensely painful arm that swelled up to many times its regular size. I looked like I had elephantiasis. Or one tuck-shop lady arm. Even today, over five years since having that procedure, I'm still trying to rectify the damage that was done. My arm is still swollen and sore; I have limited movement and whole lot of nerve damage. The fact that I can't do a downward dog in yoga without being in a heap of pain peeves me the most.

Following the limb infusion, scans showed that I was clear of cancer. However, in 2009—not even a year after going into 'remission'—I found out that the cancer was still there and had been there the whole time. Scans may not have shown up the cancer, but a biopsy of visibly growing lumps did. This time, amputation was all that my medical team could offer me, along with radiation of the shoulder and full body chemo. However, it was made clear that all of this would not cure me. It was simply intended to buy me some time. My case was deemed to be terminal.

In the midst of the horrible, harrowing angst and suffocating storm of emotions that accompanied such news, I heard a quiet yet very persistent voice inside me saying that everything was going to be okay. It told me that my arm wasn't actually the problem, that amputation was certainly not the answer, and that I would be safe and taken care of. I know now that this voice was my intuition, and it led me on a journey of research and empowerment that has ultimately saved my life.

I decided that what my doctors were offering me wasn't good enough. I wasn't ready to give my power away to some people—no matter how smart they were—who didn't really know what they were doing with it.

My family and I took matters into our own hands. I refused the doctors' offers and began searching for natural, alternative cancer treatments. The way I saw it, I had two choices: let them chase the disease around my body until there was nothing left of me to cut, zap or poison; or take responsibility for my illness and bring my body to optimum health so that it could heal itself. For me it was an easy decision.

I had a life that I loved and resented giving up. But I didn't have much choice. I knew that in order to save my life, I would have to give up pretty much everything I was familiar with. Everything that I pinned my identity to: my high-stress career, drinking, taking drugs, eating crappy food and a relationship I wasn't happy in. I swapped all of this for a lifestyle that revolved obsessively around healing.

During the time between my two diagnoses, I made the incredibly tough decision to leave my job at *Dolly*, leave

Sydney and move back to the Sunshine Coast. As much as I mourned that job, it made sense to lower the pace of my lifestyle and move somewhere more conducive to healing. I left Sydney, I left *Dolly*, and then I left the long-term relationship with the person who had been my rock through the whole recent mess. We had known each other since primary school and, while I was comfortable, something was missing.

After that string of tough decisions and leaps into unknown territory, the universe rewarded me with so many blessings. First I adopted Edie, the most beautiful little pug girl ever, and then Tallon, the love of my life (actually, probably many lives) and I started dating again (we had dated for four months when we were 19). Tallon, Edie and my incredible parents formed the most amazing support team a girl could hope for.

We became absolutely obsessed with researching cancer therapies, and the one that kept coming to the fore was Gerson Therapy. From everything I read about it, it sounded like the toughest, most labour-intensive of them all—just what I needed for my stubborn sarcoma.

Gerson Therapy is a strict and rigorous regime that involves a two-year lifestyle commitment. For two years, Gerson patients must drink 13 glasses of fresh, organic veggie juice each day—that's one on the hour, every hour. They eat a basic plant-based diet that is stripped of things like meat, salt, sugar, fat, dairy, wheat, spices, many herbs, berries, fats and other random foods that you miss like crazy. Castor oil is taken by mouth and in an enema every second day, giving you the runs and making you feel like you've got a hangover. Then there are the coffee enemas. I'm talking about a bucket of coffee that you funnel up your backside up to five times a day. Yes, that's right. It seems insane, but the coffee enemas are a crucial part of the detoxification process (and personally, my favourite part) as they help to eliminate toxins from the liver—a must when you're stirring them up with so much juice. We will get into coffee enemas a little later. Look forward to that!

I knew that, to make it through this intense therapy, I would need to get my head straight. So my first stop was the Gawler Retreat in Melbourne. Tallon and I spent 10 days there, learning how to meditate and all about the role our emotions play in disease manifestation and healing. This was such an awesome experience, but it was a holiday compared to what I was in for next.

I started my Gerson Therapy journey by going to the Gerson clinic in Mexico for three weeks. My mum came with me as my carer although, as fate would have it, she was diagnosed with breast cancer almost exactly a year into my therapy and went on Gerson herself.

The Gerson clinic is like an all-natural hospital. With the hourly juicing, five daily coffee enemas and castor oil every second day, the program is a major clean out. It's designed to reset your body, to detoxify years of built-up gunk and to flood your cells with nutrition. Nurses are at your beck and call, kitchen staff deliver juices and put on the most amazing organic vegan spreads, and doctors are there for twice-daily visits. Then, every Wednesday, Charlotte Gerson herself drives across the border from her home in San Diego to spend time with each of the patients. And did I mention she's 91 years old?

My three-week stay at the clinic wasn't the hardest part, although I missed Tallon, Edie and my Dad like crazy. It was coming home and having to float all of the elements of this therapy that was the most challenging endeavour we had to face. For two years, my life revolved around Gerson, chained to my juicer and attached to my enema bucket like it was an umbilical cord. I was forever watching the clock. I couldn't leave the house for any longer than 45 minutes, and I couldn't even sit through a whole movie without having to get up and make a juice. Going out for dinners, lunches and nights out with my friends were all out of the question.

The first year was the hardest, as I was desperately mourning my old lifestyle and just wanted the months to hurry up and be done. But in the second year something shifted. The emotional tsunamis were less frequent, I felt amazing in my body, and there was light at the end of the tunnel. Plus, this new lifestyle was just that … a lifestyle. I realised that, in order to move on with my life, I couldn't keep pining after the past. I had to let it go and make room for whatever the universe had in store for me.

In April 2012, I completed my two years of Gerson Therapy and slowly began transitioning back into the real world. I had started my blog, *The Wellness Warrior*, a week before I went to Mexico. By the time I finished Gerson Therapy, it had morphed into a business. My online tribe played a pivotal part in my journey, being there for me every single day as I went through a rollercoaster of emotions and achievements. When toxins were leaving my body and leaving me in a foul mood, my blog provided a safe sanctuary of support and love. And when I reached my two-year mark, my amazing worldwide family cheered and raised their glasses of green juice with me.

This year of 2013 marks five years since that original diagnosis. By conventional standards, I can now officially call myself a cancer survivor. But I started calling myself that on the day I decided to become an empowered participant in my healing. Now I'm a cancer thriver. I'm living proof of the body's ability to heal itself.

I can't firmly report on the status of my disease, because I no longer have scans. My previous scans weren't highlighting my cancer anyway, so I don't see much point in exposing my clean body to all of that radiation. However, I can say that I feel healthier and more vibrant than I ever have before. I have regular blood tests that my Gerson doctors are always happy with, and I will continue to monitor how my body is performing. I have 100% faith that my body knows how to heal, and I sure as heck have been giving it everything it needs to do so. Some call me crazy, but this has been the right path for me. Over the years, I've become more and more confident in my ability to know what's best for my body.

My lifestyle today is the polar opposite of what it was before the catalyst that was cancer. I don't drink alcohol; I don't take as much as a painkiller when it comes to drugs; I work from home in a job that allows me to put self care first; I'm in a relationship that makes me happier than I ever thought possible; and I have an incredible relationship with food. My insatiable appetite is still there, but I'm now blessed with the knowledge that I'm about to share with you in this book. This knowledge has opened me up to a whole world of food, nutrition and wellness that literally enables me to eat whatever I feel like eating and I never—repeat never—worry about whether I'm putting on weight. Even the most well-crafted vocabulary would not do justice to how liberating this is.

The reason I can come at you with this 'Make Peace with Your Plate' talk is because I've experienced the benefits firsthand. Not only have I healed my body, I never worry about whether the huge amounts I'm eating are making my ass grow. I no longer crave foods that I know are bad choices for my body and I no longer feel guilty after I indulge in something sweet. That's the most empowering feeling ever. I don't deprive myself of anything; I don't starve myself; I don't count calories; and I don't ever feel like I'm missing out on something. Quite the opposite, actually.

Once I started witnessing the benefits of eating such a clean, healthy and delicious diet, it was like I had a secret shared by only a select group of people. Now I know that this information isn't so much a secret but rather forgotten age-old truths that have been silenced by marketing, advertising, greed and industry propaganda. It's time we relearnt them. Are you ready? Let's do this.

MAKE PEACE WITH YOUR PLATE

PART TWO

How Did We Get Into This Mess?

CHAPTER TWO

We are mortgaging our health to pay for the pleasure of our palate. This may be hard to justify under any circumstances. But there would, at least, be a case to be made if the only way to enjoy food were to give up health. If the only food that tasted good were bad for us, we would have a tough decision to make. And some might say—to hell with health! They might come to regret it, but we could all understand the choice. But there is no such choice to be made ... Pretending that food doesn't matter to health is at best denial, at worst a serious delusion. We should not mortgage health to pay for culinary delight, any more than we should give up culinary pleasure to purchase health. We can love food that loves us back.

◦◦◦◦ Dr David Katz

We can send emails, get directions, shop on ebay from our phones, and share every element of our lives with everyone we know via social media; but for some reason we find it incredibly difficult to feed ourselves. Way, way back in the day, before phones were smart and technology paved the way for convenience, our ancestors did just fine with the task of eating. They knew what to eat, when to eat and how to eat. They didn't rely on nutritionists, dieticians, scientists, journalists or marketing hype to tell them what to chow down on; they just understood that certain foods were meant to be eaten and certain foods weren't. They used their common sense and intuition to guide them from the garden or the market to the kitchen.

Over the years, things began to change. Food was no longer just something that came out of the ground or the ocean. Suddenly food came out of a box, a jar, a packet, the freezer or a drive-through. Something else happened as well. Food was no longer just food. Instead, food became the sum of all of its nutritional parts. Suddenly we needed a whole new vocabulary just to understand how to feed ourselves. We needed a nutritionist to accompany us to the supermarket, just so we could decide between items that are fit to put in our gobs and items that aren't. Whole food was out; antioxidant-, carbohydrate-, fibre-, protein-, phytochemical- and fat- content was in. We became a nation obsessed with nutrition. But did this make us any healthier? Funnily enough, no. Quite the opposite, actually.

Michael Pollan, journalist and author of the best-selling book *In Defence of Food*, describes the ideology around our thinking about food as *nutritionism*—a pseudo-scientific way of looking at food. According to Pollan, nutritionism reduces food to its nutritional parts. We clever humans discover that a certain nutrient works wonders for our bodies and then we try to isolate it, extract it and mass reproduce it. Take carrots, for example. Carrots contain a highly beneficial nutrient called beta-carotene. Scientific types got hold of this knowledge and decided to hunt down the beta-carotene in the humble carrot, extract it and make supplements out of it. They were a little bummed when they discovered that beta-carotene supplements were a poor man's nutrient, in comparison to eating a whole carrot. Why? Because we haven't yet figured out everything that goes on in a carrot. Vegetables in their whole form house a galaxy of nutrients, enzymes and other goodness that work together to deliver amazing benefits to our bodies.

This way of looking at nutrition also divides the food world into good and evil, demonising certain nutrients while enshrining others. This could make sense if the list of 'good' guys and 'bad' guys weren't forever changing on us. Remember the days when protein was considered 'bad' and carbohydrates were 'good'? Now it is the opposite. Thanks to Dr Atkins and the slew of carb-bashers who came running to the table after him, carbs are often wrongly accused of being evil. We may be clever enough to figure out that some carbs are bad for us, but we often forget that not all carbohydrates are created equal. The same goes for fat.

The low-fat campaign began in the early 1980s and is just starting to fade out now. You know what else started around the early 1980s? The obesity epidemic and the rise of type 2 diabetes! Clearly, the science around these nutrition claims was not very sound. As soon as we were told to avoid fat at all costs, we began gorging on anything that was labelled as 'low-fat' and 'fat-free'. Never mind the amount of sugar and refined carbohydrates that were taking its place, causing us to spiral into serious health decline.

Butter was another victim of the 'low-fat' campaign. Sure, butter is an animal fat and you should by no means use it as a condiment on everything. But it's a heck of a lot better than margarine. We now know that trans fats, as found in margarine, are lethal and responsible for many diseases. On the other hand, people have been successfully eating butter for around eight or ten thousand years.

Nutritionism undermines our instincts. This modern, western style of eating has made us forget that we have things like culture, tradition and an in-built common sense to tell us what we should and shouldn't be eating. As Michael Pollan puts it, *People have eaten very well for thousands of years before they even knew what an antioxidant was, and they can do it again.*

Even bugs and mould are more in tune than us. Have you ever wondered why a loaf of white bread can sit on your counter for over a week and not be bothered by these usually hungry pests? It's because they don't recognise it as food.

The solution to wellness is very simple. We need to forget all the lingo, stay away from anything branded with a health claim (carrots don't need health claims!) and stick to the basics. Eat foods that are as close to their natural state as possible and good health will follow. Weight loss will be a given. If food can sit in your pantry for years and not go bad, don't eat it. If it contains ingredients that you can't pronounce, don't eat it. If you pick up something that your great-grandmother wouldn't recognise as food, don't eat it. It is that easy.

By eating local, organic, fresh whole foods you really can't go wrong. Your body is designed to eat food from the ground and, if you feed it accordingly, it will reward you by carrying you through a long, healthy and happy life.

∞ I DON'T BELIEVE IN COUNTING CALORIES

There are only a few things that really peeve me. One is animal cruelty, another is the incorrect use of punctuation, and the third is our modern-day obsession with counting calories. I can barely resist rolling my eyes whenever I hear someone touting the benefits of a certain food based on its calorie content, or misinformed folks who painstakingly keep diaries of their daily calorie intake. Counting and restricting calories is not effective when it comes to wellness or long-term weight loss. First of all, a 'calorie' is simply the term that is used to measure the amount of energy that we receive from food. So why are they considered evil? Calories have become victims of the 'diet' and weight loss industry and their ploy of using clever marketing to turn us all into suckers. And boy, are they succeeding! The number of people I encounter who won't eat something because it contains a certain amount of calories blows me away. Many of us have been fooled, but we are not looking any slimmer or feeling any better because of it.

It's commonly believed that, in order to lose weight, we must burn more calories than we consume. Let's consider why this is a load of bull: **Not all calories are created equal!**

Too many of us fill our diets with empty calories. This means that we're consuming calories, but not receiving any nutrients. The diet industry leads us to believe that choosing foods containing fewer calories will help us lose weight—but they don't tell us that those calories consist of sugar, preservatives, additives, and chemicals. When this is the case, the food will actually cause weight gain, not weight loss—plus, it will rob you of your health.

Let's say we had 100 calories of processed chocolate and 100 calories of broccoli. Which one is it best to eat? Or let's compare an avocado and a can of cola. A large avocado contains about 350-400 calories, a regular cola contains about 140 calories and a can of diet cola contains 0 calories. Which do you think is the healthiest? It's the avocado, of course. Avo may be high in fat, but we need fat. Fat is good for us, and fat **does not** make us fat.

Cola is an example of something that is an empty calorie: it provides us with short-term energy, but makes us feel depleted shortly after, because it brings nothing else to the table. That's not even mentioning the horrendous damage caused by artificial sweeteners, which we will get to soon. Avocado, on the other hand, contains calories that are loaded with goodness—so many vitamins, minerals and good healthy fats to keep us sustained and promote health and wellbeing.

It's also worth noting that one gram of carbohydrate contains four calories, while one gram of fat contains nine calories.

⎯ PROCESSED FOOD VERSUS WHOLE FOODS

The secret to dietary sanity lies in the adoption of one rule. Eat whole foods. Sounds easy, right? Much easier than calculating calories, weighing portions, starving yourself and locking up all of the sweets in the house. This rule is also simple to understand.

Whole food is just food that is prepared from ingredients that are as close to their natural state as possible, with all of their goodness intact. Whole foods are foods that are organic, unprocessed and unrefined. They typically do not contain added ingredients, such as sugar, salt or fat. Think of food as it was in the olden days—before we started messing around with it. Food was created perfect in the first place, so why change it?

Sticking to the whole food rule becomes a little more difficult when we go shopping. Unless you shop the outside perimeter of your supermarket, chances are you're going to be buying processed foods. Anything that's in a jar, packet, box or bottle is processed. Anything white is processed.

Processed foods do not belong in our bodies. Our bodies are extremely clever: when we try to feed them something that is processed, they recognise that they're eating something but can't figure out what it is, because it's missing so many nutrients and its molecular structure has been altered. So, to make up for the missing nutrients, our bodies tap into their own reserves and they end up taking minerals from our blood and bones. Obviously, this is not a smart move in the long run.

To embrace a whole food diet, you need to bid adieu to takeaway food, processed food, refined foods, sugars, additives, preservatives, table salt and fats. Sound tough? It's really not. It's just that, after years and years of abuse, our taste buds have basically been murdered. They have become so accustomed to overly salty, sugary, fatty and chemically-enhanced 'food' that real fodder barely registers on their radar. But I assure you that if you persist and let your taste buds be reunited with the simple, subtle flavours provided by such culinary treasures as vegetables, grains, legumes, herbs and spices, you will be pleasantly surprised by how much you enjoy them. Then, after sticking with a whole food diet for a little while, you will be rewarded by feeling and looking better than ever.

Vegetables, grains and legumes are true super foods. They are so rich in enzymes and micronutrients and are packed with a whole host of antioxidants that fight disease and slow the ageing process. They also contain considerable amounts of fibre, which helps keep your digestive system healthy, slows blood sugar responses and keeps cholesterol levels in check.

When you follow a whole food diet, you can literally eat as much as you want without worrying about your waistline. In fact, the more you eat the more nutrients your body will receive. Plus, the more you fill up on this good stuff, the less you'll feel like polluting your body with crap. You have no idea how refreshing it is to never again have to worry about the scales or being able to squeeze into your skinny jeans. After following a whole food diet for a while, your beautiful body will just find its natural groove. You'll have loads of energy, your skin will glow (once you get past the immediate detox) and you will experience a deep connection with yourself. Once you clean out the gunk, you will be able to listen to your body and understand what it really needs and wants.

This is what I'm talking about when I say that I can now eat whatever I want without worrying about weight gain. The foods that I now crave are whole foods. I never ever crave anything processed, because my body doesn't register that stuff as food. This is a far cry from the girl who used to live on microwaved dinners, microwaved pasta, microwaved rice and microwaved leftover Thai food. If it didn't come from a packet, I didn't really know what to do with it. Now, if it comes in a packet, I'm not one bit tempted to eat it.

— CHEMICALS IN OUR FOOD

There are many, many dietary theories out there that we can argue about until the Jolie-Pitt kids start adopting a multi-cultural tribe of their own. But there's one area that all clever wellness experts agree on: that the chemicals in our food are the real villains.

Packaged and processed foods certainly help save time and labour and, thanks to all the preservatives, they last forever. The inclusion of additives means we can have pasta in five minutes, noodles in two and a whole chicken dinner in fewer than ten; but what are they really feeding us? Unhealthy amounts of salt, refined sugar, bad fats and other ingredients that you'd need a scientific dictionary to decipher. They can lead to weight gain, food allergies, vitamin and mineral deficiencies, digestive disorders, skin issues, cancer and much more.

There are so many additives that I would need to make this a much larger book to list them all. So let's just go over the most common ones. Here's what you need to look for next time you analyse an ingredients label …

— ARTIFICIAL SWEETENERS

You might think you're doing your thighs a favour by choosing a 'diet' version of your favourite food or drink, but artificial sweeteners are even worse for us than regular sweeteners. They have nasty side effects, like contributing to cancer and brain disorders, because of the toxicity of their chemical breakdown in the body. Plus, in combination with other food additives like artificial colours, artificial sweeteners can have a very potent effect on nerve cells.

Neurosurgeon Dr Russell Blaylock says: *It is my opinion, and the opinion of many others, that aspartame is a dangerous neurotoxin and its use should be discouraged generally, but especially so in those harbouring neurological diseases.*

◦◦◦ REFINED SUGAR

White, highly-processed sugar is found in pretty much all processed foods (we will talk more about this in Chapter 3). Everything from tomato sauce, soup and pasta dishes to bread and bottled beverages is laced with sugar. High consumption of sugar and the corresponding elevated insulin levels can cause weight gain, bloating, fatigue, arthritis, migraines, lowered immune function, obesity, cavities and cardiovascular disease. It can also disrupt absorption of nutrients, possibly leading to osteoporosis, depression, PMS symptoms and stress.

◦◦◦ HIGH FRUCTOSE CORN SYRUP

Another crime committed by the producers of processed food is the inclusion of high fructose corn syrup in practically everything. You might be thinking: *Oh, but it's derived from corn—a vegetable—it must be okay.* That's a trap. Not only is HFCS just as addictive as white sugar, this sneaky sweetener may be even worse for our health. The corn used to make HFCS has been genetically modified and it is suspected of causing insulin resistance (believed to be a big contributor to climbing obesity rates). Corn is subsidised by the government, making it cheaper than cane sugar for use in soft drinks and processed foods, which is why you will find it lurking in pretty much anything in a packet, bottle or jar.

∞ MONOSODIUM GLUTAMATE (MSG)

Most commonly known as the flavour enhancer in Chinese food, MSG is also an ingredient in many packets found on supermarket shelves. MSG is an excitotoxin: a toxin that binds to certain receptors. For instance, it turns off the receptor that tells your brain that it's full, making you want to consume more food. Research proves that MSG causes weight gain and obesity, by damaging the appetite regulation centre in the area of the brain known as the hypothalamus, causing leptin resistance. Leptin is the hormone that controls how much a person feels like eating. The fullness, gratification and satisfaction that come from having eaten are completely lost when MSG is consumed, leading to an urge to eat that never stops. MSG supercharges the taste of food, operating on the brain and tricking it into thinking food tastes really great. MSG overstimulates the brain, causing a drug-like rush as dopamine levels rise. Side effects of MSG consumption include headaches, itchy skin and dizziness, as well as respiratory, digestive, circulatory and coronary concerns.

MSG is found in soups, sauces and gravies, and is sometimes hidden in baby food, baby formula, low-fat and no-fat milk, candy, gum and processed foods. It is applied to non-organic fruits and vegetables as a wax or pesticide. Then there's Chinese food. Even if a restaurant claims that they don't cook with MSG, I wouldn't trust them. Even if they don't add MSG themselves, many of the products they use for flavouring do contain it. Reading the ingredients label won't even keep you safe from MSG. As the public continues to catch on to the dangers of MSG, processed food manufacturers now go to great lengths to hide the presence of MSG from consumers. They often replace monosodium glutamate with MSG-containing ingredients that give no clue to its presence. They call them 'clean labels'. Manufacturers are also often less than truthful when consumers inquire about the presence of MSG in their products. MSG is also known as Accent, Ajinomoto, monosodium glutamate, monopotassium glutamate, glutamate and glutamic acid.

MSG is found and disguised in: broth, boullion, calcium caseinate, sodium caseinate, gelatin, fermented soy products (miso, shoyu, soy sauce, tamari), flavourings, hydrolysed soy products (hydrolysed plant protein, hydrolysed vegetable protein, liquid amino acids, soy protein, textured vegetable protein), kombu seaweed, malt extract, seasonings, soup stock, yeast products (autolysed yeast, yeast extract, yeast food, yeast nutrient).

Even the innocent terms 'spice' and 'natural flavour' can designate the presence of MSG.

— ARTIFICIAL COLOURS
Artificial colours are added to our foods and drinks to enhance their appearance and make them more appealing to consumers. Most are derived from coal tar and can contain up to ten parts per million of lead and arsenic yet still be generally recognised as safe by the FDA. Artificial colours can cause allergic reactions and hyperactivity and ADD in

children, and may contribute to visual and learning disorders or cause nerve damage.

∞ BHA AND BHT

BHA and BHT block the process of oil rancidity. These additives seem to affect sleep and appetite, and have been associated with liver and kidney damage, hair loss, behavioural problems, cancer, foetal abnormalities and growth retardation.

∞ SODIUM NITRATE AND NITRITE

If there was one group of foods that I would urge you to avoid at all costs it would be bacon, salami and other processed meats. They are laced with dangerous preservatives called sodium nitrate and nitrate. In the stomach, these compounds transform into cancer-causing agents called nirosamines. Noticeable side effects include headaches, nausea, vomiting and dizziness. In addition, these meats are continuously being linked to cancer, diabetes and heart disease.

∞ PESTICIDES

Pretty much all conventional foods contain pesticides. More than two billion pounds of pesticides are added to the food supply every year. Many of the pesticides used throughout the world are carcinogenic. Pesticide accumulation also undermines our ability to resist infectious organisms, may impair fertility and contributes to miscarriages and birth defects.

∞ OLESTRA (OLEAN)

Olestra is a calorie-free fat substitute used as an ingredient in snacks and chips. You may be thinking that calorie-free fat is a winner, but this additive inhibits the absorption of some vitamins and other nutrients. It can also cause diarrhoea and anal leakage. Extra fat or anal leakage? What would you prefer?

∞ PARTIALLY-HYDROGENATED VEGETABLE OIL

If you're one of the masses who fell for the margarine trap, or if you're partial to the odd biscuit or cake, you need to know about the dangers of partially-hydrogenated vegetable oil. This is made by infusing vegetable oil with hydrogen. When this occurs, the level of polyunsaturated oils (good fat) is reduced and trans fats are created. Trans fats are associated with heart disease, breast and colon cancer, atherosclerosis and elevated cholesterol.

The moral of the story is not only to read food labels carefully, but also to eat a diet that is as high in fresh whole foods as possible. You won't have to worry about deciphering the ingredients panel on a bunch of spinach!

∞ CHEMICALS ARE MAKING US FAT

If you won't refrain from eating chemicals to save your ass, maybe you will do so in order to save the size of it. In 2002, Dr Paula Baillie-Hamilton, of Stirling University in Scotland, made the observation that obesity rates have climbed in unison with chemical use over the previous 40 years. To phrase this even more simply: chemicals are making us fat.

Chemicals are everywhere. Not just in the food we eat, but also in the water we drink, the plastics we eat from, the pills we take, the products we clean with, the beauty and body care products we use, and pretty much everywhere else you look. I've said it before, but this is a drum that

I'm going to keep on banging: **We are not designed to consume chemicals!** When we do for prolonged periods of time, things are bound to get messy.

— WHY DO CHEMICALS MAKE US FAT?

There's plenty of scientific jargon that could be called upon to answer this question. For instance, the fact that they are endocrine disruptors—synthetic chemicals that mimic and interfere with natural hormones, causing weight gain. But here is an even simpler truth: our bodies are trying to protect us. Our bodies are so clever that they produce fat cells to protect our essential organs from chemical contamination. If the fat weren't there to protect us, we would be poisoned. When you look at it like this, fat is your friend. However, there is a better way. Don't consume chemicals! That way you will be healthy and at a healthy weight that is perfect for you.

The main chemical culprits to look out for are:

- BPA, found in plastic food containers, the lining of food cans and beverages

- Phthalates, used in some plastics and nail polish

- PBDEs, polybrominated diphenyl ethers (PBDEs) are a group of chemicals used as flame retardants in a wide range of products, including furniture, TVs, stereos, computers, carpets, curtains and, to a lesser degree, in some textiles, adhesives, sealants and coatings

- DDE, dichlorodiphenyldichloroethylene (DDE) is a breakdown product of the banned pesticide, DDT. We can be exposed to DDE through food, in the air and in our water

— THE MORAL OF THE STORY
Avoid chemicals as much as possible. Use glass to store your food and drinks, whenever possible, avoid drinking from plastic water bottles, use certified organic products and eat certified organic whole foods. Read the labels on everything you consume and start to be conscious of just how many chemicals you're exposing your body to. Be responsible for your body. Care about your body. And do whatever you can to live a natural, organic, clean lifestyle.

— CAN WE TRUST ENDORSEMENTS?
I used to trust endorsements from well-known health associations. If I went shopping and saw their logos or approval on a packet of pasta, a bottle of mayonnaise or a frozen microwave dinner, I would toss it in my trolley and pat myself on the back for making healthy, ass-shrinking choices for myself. Boy, was I fooled! When you walk into a fast food outlet and see that its 'food' is backed by one of the associations well-known for promoting healthy meal choices, this should tell you that something is off. Endorsements can be found on all kinds of crap convenience foods that can contain as much as 70% refined sugar. These foods can also be full of chemicals. This is because an endorsement can sometimes be purchased: a company can buy one, slap it on their products and use it as a clever marketing ploy to lure in trusting consumers.

— DECODING YOUR CRAVINGS
Back when I was working in magazines, I couldn't make it through an afternoon without picking all of the yellow, green

and orange snakes out of a bag of lollies (at least I shared the red and blue ones!). I never would have thought that, in the not too distant future, my cravings would dramatically change to a yearning for foods as crazy as green smoothies and quinoa.

Like many people, I would charge through the morning (usually powered by caffeine), but by 3pm I'd be low on energy and need a sugar hit. If my mind was swamped with thoughts, I would distract myself with a bag of chips. After every meal I craved something sweet. Can you relate? Of course you can. That's the thing about cravings—we all have them and they're all pretty similar. Why is that exactly? Because cravings actually mean more than 'It's that time in the afternoon when I need to face plant some sugar'. Who woulda thunk it?

Cravings are actually our body's way of telling us something really important. If you crave something creamy, you may be going through some emotional stuff and just need a hug or affection. Ever pigged out on a tub of ice cream when you're feeling sooky? That's your body trying to tell you something and your brain misinterpreting the message. Comfort foods like ice cream, cheeses, chocolate, cakes and cookies stimulate the production of serotonin, which has a very relaxing effect on the body. People often get upset and turn to food for 'comfort', because eating high carbohydrate comfort food floods the brain with serotonin, and serotonin can calm you down in a matter of minutes. Calm is good, cottage cheese on your ass is not. There are better ways to achieve peace, like meditation, venting to a friend, getting a massage, connecting with nature, going for a walk or relaxing in the tub with some lavender essential oil.

Another common craving is salt. If a salt craving rears its ugly head, don't be rude and slam the door in its face with some salty chips. Listen to what it is trying to tell you. A salt craving can mean that your body is lacking nutrients. Eat more fresh vegetables and whole foods and see what that does. Or, you might find that you are just thirsty and need to hydrate. Drink some water or coconut water, so that you're topping up your electrolytes.

At the end of 2009, I went on a four-week holiday to Nepal and India. We did a ten-day trek through the Himalayas and ate nothing except fried rice, followed by two weeks in India eating oily curries every day. Way back when I was living off Thai takeaway and three-minute microwave rice, my body probably would have relished the opportunity to inhale this kind of nutritionally-devoid cuisine exclusively for four weeks. However, seeing as I had been feeding my body with nutritious, organic, healing foods prior to this trip, these were the foods I craved. I was desperate for a fresh salad and juice! Your body wants what it is used to. If you constantly feed it junk, it will crave junk. If you nourish it with goodness, it will crave healthy food. The latter is the way to go.

Cravings usually precede some kind of emotional turmoil that we would rather numb ourselves out of dealing with, or they are a cry for nutrients. If you silence a craving with crap food, you can be assured of temporary relief, followed by the craving coming back even stronger than before. The only way to really get control of your cravings, whatever they might be, is to work out what your body is lacking—physically, emotionally or spiritually. Be okay about sitting with your emotions, feeling into them and letting them pass, and you won't have the need to dull the pain with food. An unpleasant emotion isn't very nice, but it won't kill you. And the only way to give it the move along and have it replaced with joy is to feel it. Also, if you follow a balanced diet that is full of fresh fruits and vegetables, grains, natural sweeteners, good fats and wholefoods, you can be sure that your cravings will subside in no time.

When we get back to basics and eat the kinds of foods that our ancestors ate, we gain back our culinary instincts. Years of consuming processed food have robbed us of this instinct. We eat for convenience and we've built up a taste for synthetic flavours, so we don't instantly recognise that our bodies don't want to consume the foods we're feeding them. If we don't throw up, we consider it a win. We don't generally link our niggling health issues back to our last meal. However, when we eliminate all of the processed foods and start eating real foods again, this instinct grows back. Then, if you've been eating clean for a little while and randomly eat something your body doesn't really want, you will know about it. You'll be sensitive to crappy foods and instantly know what you should and shouldn't be eating. I recently went to Bali for a holiday and managed to eat organic food the whole time, apart from one meal. We went to a very fancy restaurant and I ordered a Thai green curry. It went down okay and I told myself that this one conventional meal wouldn't do me any harm. My body had a different opinion though and, about an hour after I went to bed that night, I woke up feeling so sick I had to throw up. Clearly, after so many years of eating clean, my body had become completely resensitised.

— GOOD NEWS! YOU'RE NOT REALLY A BITCH!

Next time you feel depressed, unfocused, angry or lethargic, stop yourself from blaming the wrong side of the bed or the fact that you couldn't find any clean underwear, and think about whether your mood may have something to do with something you've eaten. Or something you haven't eaten.

It's hard to feel inspired and happy on a diet of processed carbohydrates, decomposing flesh and chemical, artificial junk food. Chances are you'll feel heavy and your mind will be foggy. On the other hand, eating fresh vegetables, whole grains and fruits, as well as drinking plenty of water, will make you feel alert and energised.

Processed foods deteriorate mood in two ways. Simple sugars, MSG and overrefined flour create imbalances in our system, which can lead to irritability, depression and hyperactivity. At the same time, processing removes the healthy nutrients in foods that can prevent negative moods.

According to Julia Ross, nutritional psychologist and author of the book *The Mood Cure*, junk moods come from junk foods. She writes that the current epidemic of bad moods is linked to an epidemic of deteriorating food quality.

It's kind of ironic that, when we're in a bad mood, most of us will seek comfort in a packet of chips or a block of chocolate. However, these foods are a big part of the initial problem. Salt messes with your mood by making you feel tense; and, while sugar can give you a high and make you feel energised, this feeling doesn't last long. Your blood sugar levels go up, making you feel all 'woo hoo' but, as soon as they drop again, you'll feel worse than you did to begin with. It's a vicious vending machine cycle.

This food-mood connection is maintained by neuro-transmitters—chemical messengers that relay thoughts and actions throughout the brain. Some neurotransmitters, such as serotonin, can make us feel relaxed. Others, like dopamine, have a stimulating effect. The food we eat breaks down in our digestive tract, enters our bloodstream and creates changes in the behaviour of the neurotransmitters, impacting our mood.

Think back to the last time you stuffed yourself silly on a big bowl of heavy white pasta. How did you feel after-wards? I'm guessing you weren't in the mood for running around a water park. This kind of feat usually makes you feel like undoing your top button, lying down and taking a big old nap. This is because eating carbohydrates releases serotonin and makes you feel relaxed and lazy. Eating too many carbs, or overly-processed carbs like sugar, white flour, white rice and white pasta, releases even more serotonin, causing drowsiness. Eating protein produces dopamine and norepinephrine in the brain, which makes people feel alert and full of energy. However, overeating protein can lead to tension and irritability.

Eating too much of anything can also lead to drowsiness and lethargy, because the digestive process zaps so much energy. Think about how you feel after you've just eaten someone under the table at an all-you-can-eat buffet. To handle the excess food, blood flow is directed to the stomach and away from the brain. This is why you can never handle any more stimulation than falling asleep in front of the telly.

Ways to improve your mood with food include:

- ∞ Replace processed food with fresh organic whole foods.

- ∞ Eat more soluble fibre, to slow down the absorption of sugar in your blood and lessen mood swings. Oats, brown rice, barley, apples, pears, potatoes, carrots, peas and beans are good sources. Avoid processed grains like white rice or pasta, which have been stripped of fibre and nutrients.

- ∞ Replace coffee, soft drinks and bottled juice with water, herbal tea and fresh juices.

- ∞ Avoid foods that contain artificial chemical additives.

- ∞ Eat more serotonin-rich foods like pineapples, bananas, kiwis, plums and tomatoes, as well as foods that enhance serotonin production and absorption like spirulina, beans, cereals, leafy greens and avocados.

- ∞ Eat good sources of omega-3 fats like walnuts, flax-seeds, chia seeds, hemp seeds and spirulina.

- ∞ Exercise. I know this isn't a food, but regular exercise is great for balancing your state of mind.

EXPERT WORD ⦙ DANIEL VITALIS

We're not designed to come to pieces, the way we are now as we get older. We're not meant to suffer from degenerative diseases. 100 years ago, heart disease and cancer were not issues. We don't naturally degenerate. The reason we're degenerating is because we've walked away from the natural ways for our bodies.

Daniel Vitalis is a superstar in the health and nutrition world. He teaches that invincible health is a product of living in alignment with our biological design and our role in the ecosystem. He incorporates the wisdom of ancient, time-tested, indigenous ways of life into our modern lives.

FIVE SNEAKY ELEMENTS

(THAT CAN ADD LARD TO YOUR ASS AND MIGHT TAKE YEARS FROM YOUR LIFE)

CHAPTER THREE

We have all been given a beautiful creation—our physical body. But none of us were born with an operating manual or instruction book. Most of us don't learn how to manage our energy and bodies well. We use drugs—sugar, caffeine, alcohol, adrenaline or worse—to manage our energy and moods. Most of us don't connect our behaviours and choices with how we feel every day.

We don't connect what we eat, how much we rest and sleep, how much we exercise, how much time we make for connecting with friends and community, or the kinds of media and news we watch with how we feel every day. ... Feeling fully energised and vitally healthy comes down to a very simple principle: take out the bad stuff and put in the good stuff.

∞ Dr Mark Hyman

It's fair to say that we've all been pretty gullible at some point in our lives—especially during the formative years of our youth. I don't know about you, but I ate it up when I was told that I shouldn't pee in the pool because the water would turn purple, or I shouldn't pull funny faces because the wind would change and my face would stay that way. I also didn't think to question authority when I was taught common nutrition 'truths', like the importance of dairy for calcium, meat for protein, sugar for energy, salt for minerals and bread for fibre.

When the research I was doing forced me to question the validity of these claims, I desperately wanted to be able to prove them right. I was devastated that the foods that had been my staple diet for the first 22 years of my life were turning out to be a bunch of frauds. However, as much as I wanted to ignore everything I was reading and go back to the blissful ignorance of my consumerism knowledge, I knew I couldn't betray myself in that way any longer.

So, as you read this chapter, please keep an open mind. Some of this information is not yet mainstream, but that doesn't mean that it's not true. Remember, there was also a time when doctors were promoting cigarettes and the smartest people in the world thought the Earth was flat.

∞ ELEMENT N° 1 ⦙ DAIRY

It's obvious that creamy products like ice cream, custard and cream are going to screw with your chances of looking fine and feeling svelte after a binge session, but we rarely place the same kind of blame on dairy products like milk, cheese and yoghurt. Perhaps this is because the highly affluent dairy industry pours so much money into making sure their money maker is painted in such a positive light to the public? *You need milk for strong bones!* and *Dairy, it does a body good!*—you're probably familiar with the slogans. And we can't forget about all of those incredibly beautiful celebs asking us if we've *Got milk?* while showing off their milk moustaches. The truth is that all of this pro-dairy propaganda is bull. We don't need dairy to complete a healthy diet. In fact, dairy could be responsible for many of your unexplained health and weight issues. Here's why ...

⸺ Humans aren't made to digest cow's milk

Dairy is nature's perfect food—but only if you're a calf says Dr Mark Hyman. Humans are the only animals to drink the milk of other species and to drink milk at all past infancy. Each mammalian species has its own 'designer' milk, and cow's milk is no exception. Its composition is very different to human milk. For example, cow's milk contains on average three times the amount of protein in human milk. This creates metabolic disturbances in humans that have detrimental bone health consequences. Cow's milk is also designed to rapidly fatten up baby cows by filling up all of their four stomachs.

⸺ Dairy can cause calcium deficiency

Say what?! It turns out all those ads telling us that the calcium in dairy will give us strong bones were all a load of baloney. Countries with the lowest rates of dairy consumption (like those in Africa and Asia) have the lowest rates of osteoporosis. The consumption of dairy actually contributes largely to a deficiency in calcium in the body. Animal protein (found highly in dairy) increases the acid load in the body. In order to neutralise that acid and bring the body back to an alkaline state, the body searches its own reserves for an alkaline mineral. Enter calcium. But this calcium ends up being pulled from our bones, in turn leading to bone-weakening conditions like osteoporosis. Dairy may contain calcium, but it is of no use to our bodies. Shocking, isn't it? It's like finding out that the Easter Bunny isn't real.

∞ Excessive consumption of Dairy can lead to heart disease

Some dairy products are high in saturated fats and trans fats. These fats are strongly associated with the development of heart disease (and cottage cheese on your thighs).

∞ The antibiotics issue

Dairy cows (and all livestock) are pumped with antibiotics to prevent diseases that would otherwise be rampant, due to poor living conditions on factory farms. They are also fed processed grains and genetically-modified corn that are not really meant for their consumption.

∞ Dairy is bad for your digestive system

Humans lose the enzyme needed to digest lactose (the sugar found in milk) between the ages of two and five. When undigested, the sugars from dairy end up in the colon, where they begin to ferment, producing gas that can cause cramping, bloating, nausea, flatulence and diarrhoea. Dairy is also known to cause asthma, allergies, strep throat, tonsillitis, ear infections, pimples/ acne, weight gain, and excessive mucus and phlegm.

∞ **Dairy can increase your cancer risk**
Cows are like humans, in that they only produce milk when pregnant. To counteract this problem, dairy farmers inject their milking cows with a genetically-engineered form of bovine growth hormone (rBGH). A man-made or synthetic hormone used to artificially increase milk production, rBGH also increases levels of the insulin-growth factor 1 (IGF-1) in the blood of those who drink it. And higher levels of IGF-1 are linked to several cancers. The Harvard School of Public Health assessed that: ...*high intake can increase the risk of prostate cancer and possibly ovarian cancer.* The book entitled *The China Study* by T Colin Campbell is also an excellent source, if you want to read more on this.

∞ ELEMENT N° 2 ⦙ **FLESH**
Let's get one thing straight before you judge the content of this section by its title. I'm not about to tell you to give up meat. I don't actually believe that **everyone** should give up meat. I'm not here to judge whether you're an omnivore, vegetarian, pescetarian or vegan. Eating meat is a personal decision, and I don't have the right or the knowledge to say whether it's a good choice for you or not. I've seen many people whose health has declined after cutting meat from

their diets, and I've also seen many people whose health has astronomically thrived—mine included (for now, anyway). The thing is that we're all made differently and it's up to us individually to honestly discover whether our bodies work better on purely plants, or with a little meat in the mix. I encourage you to experiment with this and pay attention to how your body responds. Don't remain hell-bent on one way of eating, just because you're afraid to stray from the label it awards you. Also, don't be afraid of trying something new, just because it's unknown to you.

Now that I've made all of that clear, I'm still going to stand by my opinion that most of us eat far too much meat. Even if you are a meat eater, you do not need to eat meat three times a day, seven days a week. When you finish reading this section, you'll understand why. If you do decide that you would still like to include meat in your diet, perhaps you'll just need to reduce your intake. Instead of having the majority of your plate covered by animal, with salad and veggies as a side dish, switch it around. Make plants the main attraction and just have meat as a condiment. Also, make sure you have plenty of meat-free meals, or even meat-free days because …

— **Meat is difficult to digest**

Because meat contains absolutely no fibre, it creates a lot of work for your small intestines. It can take up to three days for meat to pass through your system. Your small intestines have a lot of trouble pushing the meat through. It can get stuck in there, putrefying and creating acidity. It also causes blockages, so that other food gets stuck in your intestines. It's pretty gross when you think about it. If you have poor digestion, your body won't absorb the nutrients it needs from your food. (We will talk about this more in a later chapter.)

Meat is full of antibiotics

It's highly doubtful that the meat you see on your dinner plate came from an animal that had been allowed to roam free in a big grassy paddock. According to *Animals Australia*, 85-90 per cent of our meat comes from factory farms. To cope with the western world's mass demand for meat, traditional Old MacDonald-style farms have been replaced by corporate, money-hungry factory farms. In a factory farm, chickens, pigs, turkeys and cows are treated like machines, instead of living, feeling individuals. Unnaturally large numbers of animals are confined closely together with no grass or vegetation. Cattle feedlots generally contain thousands of animals in one place, while many egg-laying businesses house one million or more chickens. The animals are crammed in and forced to live in their own faeces, urine and vomit. The conditions in which they are kept are so poor that they are pumped with antibiotics, so that they don't die from the myriad of diseases they are sure to catch. To give you an idea of the level of antibiotics administered to animals in the US: about three million pounds of antibiotics are given to humans each year whereas, by comparison, *The Union of Concerned Scientists (UCS)* calculated that 24.6 million pounds are fed to farmed animals for non-therapeutic uses.

Because of poor living conditions and the fact that they are fed an unnatural diet of cheap, low-grade grain and corn, these animals are often very sick. Antibiotics are used to keep them alive, just long enough to make it to slaughter.

∞ Meat is full of hormones

When you compare the size of a chicken today at 47 days with a chicken from the 1950s at 68 days, you can see we've been tampering with nature. Chickens, turkeys, pigs and cows are pumped with growth hormones, so that they get really big really fast. To keep up with the demand for meat, factory farmers are now resorting to unnatural measures. They have caught on to the fact that, if their animals grow faster, they can produce more animal products—never mind the damage this does to the animal or the health of the person who will eventually eat it. While chicken meat producers in Australia stopped giving chickens growth hormones in the 1960s, the selective breeding of chickens has resulted in drastic changes to the natural growth process. These poor animals now grow so fast their bones and muscles don't have time to develop properly. They're crippled under the weight of their own bodies. After the animal is killed and prepped for your dinner plate, the hormones stay in the flesh and are passed directly on to you. Excess hormones—especially second-hand hormones—have been linked to many cancers, including breast and prostate.

Plant protein versus animal protein

When I'm done with this spiel, the question that usually follows is, 'But where do you get your protein from?!' Thanks to societal conditioning, it's a common belief that we only get adequate amounts of protein from a meat-based diet. This is totally false. You don't actually need to eat meat to consume enough protein to be healthy! It's very easy for a vegan and vegetarian diet to meet the recommendations for protein, by simply including enough food from a variety of sources like vegetables, beans, grains, nuts, and seeds. Popeye, being partial to green leafy vegetables like spinach, had the right idea. Each and every plant food contains complete protein in varying amounts. Some foods like spirulina, lentils, chickpeas, quinoa, broccoli, asparagus, bamboo shoots and Brussels sprouts are very high in protein. Believe it or not, some actually contain a higher percentage of protein (as a percentage of total calories) than beef, milk or eggs. Think about the largest land animals we have, like elephants and gorillas. They are all plant eaters!

Many people are also under the misconception that you need a lot of protein in your diet to be healthy. Protein is certainly an essential nutrient and plays many key roles in the way our bodies function and repair; but we don't need huge quantities of it. Our obsession with following a high protein diet could do us more harm than good. High protein diets have been linked to several health issues, including osteoporosis, kidney stones, reduced kidney function, gout and arthritis, as well as cancer of the breast, prostate, pancreas, colon, rectum and uterus. Rather than worrying about not getting enough protein, we should be more concerned about our source of protein. If it's predominantly animal derived, not only are you more than likely getting too much, you're also getting cholesterol and saturated fat and missing out on the fibre, carbohydrates, vitamins and minerals that are only available from plant food.

The rules for eating meat

It's totally fine if you're not keen to give up meat all together. I'm not asking you to become a passionate vegan, if you don't want to. I'm just asking you to change the quality and quantity of the meat you eat.

∞ Rule 1

Meat should not be consumed more than once per day, and ideally only three times per week.

∞ Rule 2

Only buy meat that is organic, hormone-free, grass-fed and grass-finished. Grill your butchers about where they source their meat, or ask if you can visit the farm yourself. A farmer with nothing to hide is a farmer you can trust.

What about fish?

Animals from the sea are much easier on our digestive system than land animals; and fish is a great source of omega-3s. However, fish falls into two main categories: farmed and wild. Farmed fish are raised in much the same environment as factory-farmed animals. They are crammed into confined spaces and forced to survive in atrocious conditions. The enormous amount of faeces in their enclosures leads to rampant outbreaks of parasites and disease. In order to keep the fish alive in such unhealthy conditions, large quantities of antibiotics and other chemicals are poured into the water. Farmed fish are fed a tasty diet of junk grains, soy meal, corn gluten meal, chemicals and neurotoxins. Everything the fish endures is consumed by you, when you eat it!

Wild-caught fish are a little better, but still not great. Our environment is now polluted to the extent that our waterways and our seafood are contaminated with toxins like mercury, which is the second most toxic element on Earth after radiation. If you're going to eat seafood, it's best to choose small fish, like sardines and whiting. Check online for a full list of seafood that contains the most and least amounts of mercury.

What about eggs?

Just as an unborn human baby is affected by everything its mother eats and experiences, the same goes for a chicken egg. All the hormones, antibiotics and toxins that are consumed by the mother chook are absorbed into the egg.

If you think you're dodging this bullet by buying only 'free-range' or 'cage-free' eggs, think again. 'Cage-free' simply means the birds are not in cages. They are still exposed to all of the same horrific living conditions; they are fed the same unnatural diet; and only manage to stay alive by being given a steady stream of antibiotics. 'Free-range' just means the birds have access to the outside. What they don't tell you is that the area they are briefly allowed access to is no bigger than the size of an A4 piece of paper. As Jonathan Safran Foer writes in his brilliant book, *Eating Animals: I could keep a flock of hens under my sink and call them free-range.*

If you're going to include eggs in your diet, keep them to a minimum (they are still high in cholesterol and have an acid effect on the body) and make sure you only buy organic. Better still, source your eggs from a farm that you are familiar with or raise your own chickens at home.

∞ ELEMENT N° 3 ‖ SUGAR

Sugar is like crack. It sends you on the same destructive ride of highs, crashes and uncontrollable cravings that you get when you're into drugs. Only this drug of choice is socially acceptable—which means we can get our fixes all day, every day. No-one will look twice, unless you're caught trying to shake a bag of lollies out of the office vending machine. Not only is sugar highly addictive and does not provide your body with any goodness whatsoever, it actually robs you of nutrients.

White sugar is so highly processed we can hardly even call it food anymore. It's been tampered with and turned into something so artificial that our bodies don't really know what to do with it. When we shovel something that contains white sugar into our mouths, our bodies get confused. They recognise that they've eaten something but, because sugar offers absolutely no nutritional benefit, our body offers up the missing nutrients, leaching them from the blood and bones. This is why white sugar has been dubbed an 'anti-nutrient', as it actually takes nourishment from the body. This can lead to tooth decay, bone loss, depression and weak blood. On top of that, white sugar suppresses your immune system, causes crazy mood swings, has been associated with cancer, contributes to diabetes, dulls your brain and makes you fat.

Sugar literally stops your brain from registering that you're full. Research has shown that eating sugar dulls the brain's mechanism for telling you when to stop eating. Sugar blunts the brain's anorexigenic oxytocin system, which is responsible for letting you know that you're full. When this system fails, you continue to gorge.

I'm not just talking about the white (or brown) sugar that you spoon into your cup of tea or sprinkle on your breakfast. Sugar is hiding in almost all processed foods, drinks, sauces, spreads and anything else that is manufactured. Human beings love sweet flavours, so food manufacturers are clever enough to cash in on that.

∞ ELEMENT N° 4 ⦚ SALT

Table salt or 'white' salt is refined and processed to the point where it is completely devoid of all the nutrients and minerals that are found naturally in salt. Like white sugar, white processed salt will rob nutrients from your body, rather than provide them. A high-in-processed-salt diet will cause your body to retain fluid and be acidic—ultimately creating a breeding ground for problems like heart disease, kidney disease, osteoporosis and cancer. Processed table salt is the evil substance that is added to all canned, bottled, packaged, processed and takeaway foods.

What about sea salt?

Even though real unprocessed sea salt does contain minerals and nutrients that are beneficial to the body, the term 'sea salt' is essentially meaningless. Virtually all salt comes from the sea, and white processed salt can still be called 'sea salt', even though it is completely devoid of all sea minerals. The way you can tell if the sea salt you are buying is the goods is to look at the colour. If it's pure white, chances are it's been processed. Truly natural salts are usually sandy or brownish in colour.

∞ ELEMENT N° 5 ⦙ REFINED GRAINS

There's a big difference between grains that are whole and grains that are refined. Sadly, the most prominent difference is that refined grains are the ones that are most favoured in terms of appearance, taste and convenience. Most people will choose white rice over brown rice and white pasta over brown pasta any day, because this is what they're used to. And because it's still a grain, many people are fooled into thinking that it's acceptable to eat.

The truth is that refined grains convert straight into sugar when we eat them, in the form of glucose. As soon as you start chewing a refined grain, it morphs into sugar and starts doing damage.

Grains are refined to lengthen shelf life and improve their aesthetic appeal. Our first point of caution should be the 'longer shelf life' portion of their so-called benefits. If mice and insects won't even eat the bread, shouldn't that tell us something? Next time you're at the supermarket, pick up a loaf of typical white bread, flip it over and read its list of ingredients. You may be surprised to learn that most of what is listed can hardly be classed as food.

Remember the ol' rule: **if it's not food, don't eat it.** I've had a cheeseburger sitting in my dining room for over a year and the bun still looks almost identical to how it looked when I brought it home. No insects or rodents have tried to eat it and it's not mouldy. It's a gross experiment, but I'm leaving it there to scare our houseguests away from processed foods and refined grains.

The trouble with dairy, flesh, refined sugar, refined salt and refined grains is not only that they are all doing their bit to cause issues with your health. When they work together, things can be disastrous. And, let's be honest, the five above elements are staples of the modern, western diet. It doesn't matter how resilient we are, if we continuously eat these things, sooner or later something is going to show up. And I don't just mean on the scales or in the mirror, even though each of these five contribute massively to muffin tops and cellulite. Podgy areas and bad skin are merely symptoms of underlying health concerns. Health concerns, if left unchecked, can manifest into serious debilitating and life-threatening disease. We don't want that now, do we?

EXPERT WORD ⦚ DR FRANK LIPMAN

My philosophy on food is to eat as close to nature as possible. I believe that once we start altering the foods they become problems. Gluten, for instance, is an altered food. Wheat is the main gluten grain that we eat the most of and it's the grain with the most gluten in it. The wheat today is very different to the wheat of our ancestors, so we're eating an altered grain. It's a transformed product of genetic research. Dairy is altered—it's been homogenised and pasteurised. Meat—if you're eating organic and grass-fed meat I don't have a problem with that, but most meat is factory-farmed and factory-farmed meat is really bad for you. My philosophy, as a general rule, is to eat as close to nature as possible. Eat unaltered foods, and within that context there's also sugar. Most people eat too much sugar; so, if you want sugar, get it from fruits.

Chemicals on food are a major problem. They're a major issue in causing us sickness and obesity. The chemicals in our food are connected to the obesity epidemic. It's not just how much you eat and the sugars and the bad fats; but a lot of it has to do with the chemicals in the food as well. The chemicals are endocrine disruptors, so they affect your insulin metabolism amongst other hormones and can lead to obesity and diabetes.

Dr Frank Lipman is a pioneer and internationally-recognised expert in the field of integrative medicine. He is the founder and director of the *Eleven-Eleven Wellness Center* in New York City. He is also the 'go-to' medicine man for many Hollywood big names.

POWER TO THE PLANTS

You're probably pretty depressed right about now. If you're like the majority of the modern population, I've just gone through and ruled out everything that makes up your staple diet. I have great news though. There's a whole other world of food out there that is healthy, harmless and ... wait for it ... delicious. Your fridge and cupboards won't be bare for long!

No, I haven't been smoking the wacky weed. Healthy, wholesome, nourishing food can also be delicious. There's no way I would have been able to stick to such a clean diet for so long if it wasn't tasty as well. As I've said before, we were given all of our taste buds for a reason. We are supposed to enjoy good food. Our only problem is that our idea of good food became twisted as advertising and marketing and got into our heads.

The first rule for eating a healthy diet is to eat whole foods. If Mother Nature made it, you're pretty safe. The second rule is to load up your plate with plants. Even if you do choose to eat meat, plants should be the star performers during your meal times. This is because plants (as in vegetables, fruits, whole grains, legumes, beans, nuts and seeds) are the keepers of everything we need to thrive and survive. They are packed with vitamins, minerals, enzymes and antioxidants. Without plants, we would literally not be able to survive. Not very well, and not for very long anyway. Plants are our life force. They are also the source of our youth, vitality, vigour and energy. From a personal perspective, ever since I began the vegetarian transition, my mind has gained an unexplainable sense of clarity, my eyes are brighter, my skin is brighter (despite the odd detox breakout) and my body has effortlessly found and settled in to its ideal weight. Put simply, I work better on plants.

Seriously, I can't believe how easy it was and how good I feel as a result. It's unbelievable how much lighter I feel, both literally and figuratively. Not only do I never worry about my weight, but it's like my body has been relieved of all the gunk and crap that had been weighing it down. I owe all of this to eating a proper plant-based diet. I say 'proper' here, because going vegetarian or vegan isn't the only aspect of all of this, although it plays a major part. No animals go into producing salt, sugar, white flour and packets of chips. Again, the key is eating 'whole' plant-based foods.

∞ GOING GREEN

I'm going to say something really radical right now. Kale changed my life. If you don't know what kale is, then google it. Just kidding, I'll tell you what it is. Kale is a plant; a vegetable, to be more precise. But it's the type of vegetable that makes it so special. Kale is a leafy green vegetable, and leafy greens are like magic. Forget all of the fads; these guys are the real superfoods.

This group doesn't just end with kale. It also includes spinach, silver beet, Swiss chard, broccoli, cabbage, collards, brussels sprouts, watercress, romaine lettuce, etc.

It's the extremely rich chlorophyll content that gives these veggies their green colour. The molecular structure of chlorophyll is very similar to that of human blood. Studies show that, when chlorophyll is consumed, the production of haemoglobin in blood is increased. Higher amounts of haemoglobin in the bloodstream mean more oxygen-rich blood, the first and most important element that cells need to thrive. So green superfoods are incredibly alkalising, will help keep your body young and protect you from disease and illness. They also boast high amounts of easily digestible nutrients, enzymes, fat burning compounds, vitamins, minerals, proteins, protective photochemicals and healthy bacteria that all help you build cleaner muscles and tissues as well as aid your digestive system.

━ GIVE ME A 'PEE' FOR PH

Unless you paid attention in Science class, you probably scratch your head at the mention of the term 'alkalising'; but it's actually one of the simplest ways to get a grasp on the health of your body. Whether your body is acidic or alkaline is determined by your pH reading. Your body needs to have a pH reading of between 7.35 and 7.45 in order to be alkaline. A reading below 7 (which is neutral) means your body is acidic. An acidic body does not absorb vitamins, minerals and other nutrients and has a reduced ability to repair cells. Acidity also prevents the blood from carrying oxygen. Poor health thrives in an acidic, oxygen-deprived environment. However, if your body is alkaline, it will thrive and heal readily.

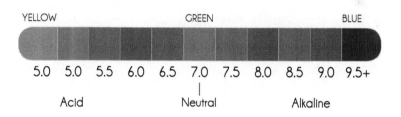

It's a whole lot easier to be too acidic than it is to be too alkaline. Acidity is caused by eating crap food, drinking alcohol, taking drugs (pharmaceutical and recreational), lack of sleep, not getting enough exercise and constantly being stressed out. Alkalinity is achieved by eating a diet that is high in clean, organic, plant-based whole foods and maintaining a calm and peaceful inner environment. Now do you see why most of us are leaning towards the acidic side? To break it down even further for you, here is a list of the most common acidic foods and the most common alkaline foods.

— THE ACID/ALKALINE DIVISION
Alkaline Foods

- Green veggies
- Green superfoods (chlorella, spirulina, barley grass powder, marine phytoplankton, wild blue-green algae, wheatgrass)
- Lemons, limes and grapefruits (they are acidic prior to being consumed, but have an alkalising affect on the body)
- Root vegetables (potatoes, sweet potatoes, turnips etc)
- Avocados
- Almonds, brazil nuts, sesame seeds, flaxseeds
- Grains such as quinoa, wild rice, millet, buckwheat, amaranth
- Raw tomatoes
- Sprouts
- Seaweed
- Raw apple cider vinegar
- Lentils and other beans
- Herbal teas (green tea, white tea, dandelion tea)

Acidic Foods

- Alcohol
- Animal protein (all meat including chicken and fish, eggs, dairy)

- Drugs, cigarettes and heavy metals (aluminium, mercury, cadmium, radium, arsenic)
- Pesticides, herbicides (including those sprayed on foods)
- Preservatives, additives, chemicals
- All processed foods (anything in a bottle, box, jar or packet)
- Table salt
- Artificial sweeteners
- Coffee (including decaf), black tea
- Refined grains, wheat and oats (brown rice and oats are mildly acidic; white rice, white bread and white pasta are highly acidic)
- Soy sauce
- Processed soy products
- Some legumes like chickpeas, black beans and soy beans are slightly acidic
- Yeast and vinegar

TESTING YOUR PH

The most common way to test your pH is with your bodily fluids—either your saliva or your urine; but I've found urine to be more accurate. A blood test is not the way to go, because your blood must always remain alkaline. As I mentioned earlier, if your blood is in danger of becoming acidic, our bodies are so clever they will resort to taking alkaline minerals from their own reserves to replenish the blood.

Testing your pH is so easy that you can do it at home. All you need to do is pee on some paper! Do this:

1. Head out to the pharmacy to buy some pH paper.
2. Pee on the piece of pH paper.
3. Wait about 20 seconds and compare the colour of the paper with the colour of the scale on the pH paper dispenser. You want it to fall somewhere between 6.8 and 7.5.
4. The best times to test your pH are on your second pee of the day (your first may give an inaccurate reading, due to metabolic processes from the night before), before meals or at least one hour after eating.

To determine your accurate pH, test yourself several times a day for about a week. At the end of the week, analyse all of your results and find your average. This is your body's pH level.

DRINK YOUR VEGGIES
The best, easiest, quickest and often tastiest way to load your body up with beautifying plants is by drinking them. Juices and smoothies are like precious elixirs of life—your best ally when it comes to saying hello to health and beauty and saying goodbye to illness and excess weight. Drinking veggie juices and smoothies is like delivering a big shot of enzymes, oxygen and vitamins straight into your blood stream.

JUICING OR BLENDING: WHICH IS BETTER?
Juices and smoothies serve two different, yet equally important, roles in our wellness regime. I'm fiercely loyal to my juicer—having drunk 13 juices a day while on Gerson

Therapy, the thing practically saved my life. But smoothies are pretty great as well.

When we juice our veggies, we're removing the indigestible fibre and making the nutrients more readily available to the body in much larger quantities than if you were to eat the fruits and vegetables whole. When you drink fresh veggie juices, your body is being soaked in nutrients, without having to use up any of its precious energy. Sitting down to eat five large carrots and one large apple would take a heck of a lot longer to do than if you were to juice those suckers. I can't imagine it would be as enjoyable or tasty either.

Unlike juices, smoothies still contain all of the fibre from the vegetables and fruits; however the blending process breaks the fibre apart and makes it easier to digest. It also makes the nutrients trapped inside the cell walls of the veggies readily available to our bodies. Smoothies are more filling and generally faster to make than juice, so they can be great to drink first thing in the morning as your breakfast, or for snacks throughout the day. Plus, you can pimp your smoothies with things like superfoods, nut milks and nut butters to really ramp up their super powers.

∞ JUICING AND BLENDING RULES!

∞ If you're juicing starchy veggies like carrots, beetroots, broccoli and zucchini, don't combine them with any other fruit besides green apple. It will only mess with your digestive enzymes. In his book *Food Combining Made Easy*, Dr Herbert Shelton explains that starchy foods have to be eaten alone, because starches are digested with enzymes that are different from those used by any other food group. Combining starchy foods with fruit may cause fermentation and gas. However, Dr Shelton found that green leafy veggies combine well with pretty much everything.

— Keep the sugar content of your juices and smoothies to a minimum, by only adding a small amount of fruit. Don't add any more than one piece of fruit, like a banana to a green smoothie or a green apple to a green juice.

— Try to drink your juice or smoothie straight away. For juices, light and air will destroy much of the nutrients after just 15 minutes. Smoothies last a little longer, but I wouldn't wait for any longer than a day or two. If you can't drink a smoothie straight away, transfer to a dark airtight glass jar (like a Mason jar) until you're ready.

— Clean your equipment after each use. Otherwise pulp will get caught in the machine and oxidise making your next juice all gross.

— THE RIGHT EQUIPMENT

To get the greatest benefit from your juices and smoothies, it's important to use the right equipment. A good juicer and a good blender are two of the best appliances you can add to your kitchen.

Juicers

Cheaper, centrifugal juicers introduce heat and oxygen, which destroy the much-needed nutrients in your fruits and vegetables. They also struggle when it comes to juicing greens. While it may cost you a bit more initially, a premium masticating, cold-press juicer will produce a superior-quality juice and allow you to extract more from your fruits and vegetables, saving expense in the long term. The machines themselves will also generally last longer. In contrast to the rough extraction of centrifugal juicers, mastication or cold-press juicers compress fruit and vegetables to 'squeeze' out their juice. You wouldn't think that the taste of juice could vary so much—but when it comes out of a top quality juicer, it's like drinking liquid sunshine!

My top three juicers:

Best: The Norwalk Juicer

This baby is the Rolls-Royce of juicers. It's made to order in California and produces by far the best-tasting juice I've ever tried. It works with a two-step process, by first grinding the veggies and spitting the pulp into a cloth bag. The bag is then placed into the 'press' section, and all of the juice is squeezed out. The result is all juice and no fibre. The only downside of the *Norwalk* is that it's super expensive (in the thousands)—especially when you live on the other side of the world to California and have to factor in the cost of shipping and customs.

Tip: Check online to see if anyone is selling one second-hand.

Better: The Angel

Made entirely from stainless steel, this gorgeous-looking machine is a twin gear juicer, that produces juice by pressing produce between two interlocking roller gears. The juice is slowly squeezed out and the pulp is gently discarded. This juicer is powerful enough to handle fibrous veggies and you'll also be able to have fun, making nut butters and fruit ice creams.

Good: The Hurom

This is a masticating juicer that works by grinding your produce into a pulp, much like the way our teeth grind when we chew. This means that the process is slower and gentler, retaining nutrients and extracting more juice from the pulp.

∞ BLENDERS

A decent blender is going to make life in the kitchen that much more enjoyable. Not only are they a must for smoothies that are smooth rather than chunky, a good blender will also enable you to make nut milks, nut cheeses, nut cheesecakes, and other raw desserts. It's also important to have a blender that is gentle on your produce and doesn't heat up the enzymes as it's pulling apart the fibres.

My top three blenders:

Best: Vitamix

A *Vitamix* is a kitchen luxury; but there's a good reason for it's high price tag—it's the best. No other blender compares to the power and speed of this machine. I highly recommend saving up for one! You won't regret it.

Better: Blendtec
Blendtec is slightly cheaper than *Vitamix*, and some people prefer it as a machine too. The jug is square at the base and easy to clean, and it does its job—blending stuff until it's smooth.

Good: OmniBlend
Cheaper again, the *OmniBlend* is a great buy if you're serious about blending, but don't want to commit to the pricier machines just yet.

When on the go: Tribest Personal Blender
For a machine so small, it's super powerful. It's small enough to fit in a travel bag, and so convenient that you blend your smoothie right in the cup you drink it from.

∞ GREEN SUPERFOODS
If you really want to go the extra mile in the green drink department, you can get all creative by throwing some green superfoods into the mix. I'm talking grasses and algae. I used to think that grass was something you mowed or smoked; but it turns out that grasses are actually incredibly good for us to churn up and drink. And algae is much more than something that gets stuck to the bottom of a boat. Here's why ...

∞ Wheat grass
Super alkalising and excellent for promoting healthy blood, wheat grass normalises the thyroid gland to stimulate your metabolism. It also assists with digestion and promotes weight loss, due to its high enzyme

content and cleansing effect. It's best to have fresh, juiced wheat grass rather than the powdered stuff.

∞ Barley grass

Barley grass has 11 times more calcium than cow's milk, five times more iron than spinach and seven times more vitamin C and bio-flavonoids than orange juice. It contains significant amounts of vitamin B12, which is very important in a vegetarian diet. Barley grass juice promotes anti-viral activity and neutralises heavy metals in the blood, eg mercury.

∞ Wild blue-green algae

Wild blue-green algae is a phyto-plankton and contains virtually every nutrient. It has 60 per cent protein content and is one of the best-known food sources of beta-carotene, B vitamins and chlorophyll. It has been shown to improve brain function and memory, strengthen the immune system and help with viruses, colds and flu.

∞ Spirulina

Spirulina is the world's highest source of complete protein (65%) and it provides a vast array of minerals, trace elements, phytonutrients and enzymes. No green smoothie is complete without the inclusion of spirulina. The powder is best, but it also comes in capsules and tablets. My favourite brand is Green Nutritionals' *Hawaiian Pacifica*, because it is the only powder I've found that doesn't taste like a pond.

∞ Chlorella

Chlorella contains a complete protein profile: all the B vitamins, vitamin C, vitamin E and many minerals. It is amazing for the immune system, for reducing cholesterol and preventing the hardening of the arteries (a precursor to heart attacks) and strokes. Yaeyama Pacifica from Green Nutritionals is my favourite brand.

∞ Marine phytoplankton

According to eccentric superfood expert, David Wolfe, marine phytoplankton is the number one food on the planet. It grows in the ocean and produces more oxygen than all the forests combined times three! It's a complete protein source, contains EPA and DHA, is 100% pure without contaminants and is one of the highest mineral and anti-oxidant foods.

∞ OTHER SUPERFOODS

Smoothies don't have to be limited to greens! Add any of these powerhouses to your drink to give it some serious nutrition kick:

∞ Cacao

This is chocolate that is good for you! Do I really need to go on? It's chocolate in its pure form—before heat and additives destroyed it. Cacao is the highest antioxidant food on the planet, the number one source of antioxidants, magnesium, iron, manganese and chromium. It is also extremely high in PEA, theobromine (cardiovascular support) and anandamide (the 'bliss chemical'). Raw chocolate improves cardiovascular health, builds strong bones, is a natural aphrodisiac, elevates mood and energy and increases longevity.

⸺ Maca

Maca root powder increases energy, endurance, strength and libido. It contains more than 10% protein, nearly 20 amino acids and includes 7 essential amino acids.

⸺ Chia seeds

Chia seeds are thought to be the richest provider of omega-3 fatty acids and soluble dietary fibre that we can add to our diets. The protein content is enough to meet the full amount of daily protein required in our diet. This tiny seed also provides us with vitamins B, C, E and calcium.

⸺ Hemp seeds

Hemp seeds are packed with 33% pure digestible protein, and are rich in iron, amino acids and vitamin E, as well as omega-3s and GLA.

⸺ Goji berries

Goji berries contain 18 kinds of amino acids, including all 8 essential amino acids, up to 21 trace minerals, high amounts of antioxidants, iron, polysaccharides, B and E vitamins, as well as many other nutrients.

⸺ Bee pollen

Bee pollen is the most complete food found in nature. It contains nearly all B vitamins, especially vitamin

B-9 (folate) and all 21 essential amino acids, making it a complete protein.

∞∞∞ Camu berry

Camu berry is the highest vitamin C source on the planet. It's great for rebuilding tissue, purifying blood, as well as enhancing immunity and energy. Camu berry is one of the best anti-depressants, immune builders and eye-nourishing superfoods in the world.

∞∞∞ Aloe vera

The gel of the aloe vera plant can be used internally and externally for amazing benefits. When applied topically, it is great for healing wounds, moisturising skin and soothing burns. Internally, it has a lubricating effect on the joints, brain, nervous system and the skin. It is also amazing for digestion, helps increase nutrient absorption, is effective at killing yeast (candida), enhances the presence of friendly bacteria, normalises pH levels and acts as a prebiotic.

∞∞∞ Coconut

I love everything about the coconut. It is probably my favourite member of the culinary world. Coconut oil is the healthiest fat on the planet (yes, even though it is saturated); and coconut water is super high in electro-lytes and potassium.

∞∞∞ Lucuma

Pronounced loo-koo-mah, this Peruvian fruit is known as "nature's caramel". When eaten in its powdered form (which is how we generally find it) it gives a yummy caramel taste to raw desserts, baking, and smoothies. It's also an awesome natural sweetener, being low in sugars and low on the glycemic scale, but boasting a subtly sweet flavour. Nutritional properties include antioxidants like beta carotene, complex carbohydrates, fibre, vitamins such as niacin (B3) and minerals such as zinc, calcium and iron.

∞ Sea vegetables

These include kelp, dulse, nori, hijiki, bladderwrack, chlorella, etc. Rich in life-giving nutrients drawn in from the ocean and sun, sea vegetables help remove heavy metals, detoxify the body of radioactive iodine, provide numerous trace minerals, regulate immunity and decrease the risk of cancer. Seaweeds benefit the entire body and are especially excellent for the thyroid, immune system, adrenals and hormone function.

∞ Medicinal mushrooms

Including reishi, chaga, cordyceps, maitake, shiitake and lion's mane, mushies are high in polysaccharides and super immune-enhancing components.

∞ WHY ORGANIC?

If organic farming is the natural way, shouldn't organic produce just be called 'produce' and make the pesticide-laden stuff take the burden of an adjective?

∞ Ymber Delecto

Whenever I mention how important all of these plants and whole foods are, I am, of course, talking about the organic versions. To me, conventional produce is so nutritionally compromised that it's hard to even have it sitting on the same metaphorical shelf as the organic stuff.

Not only has conventional produce been sprayed with chemicals like pesticides, herbicides and fungicides, it's also been grown in soil that is seriously depleted of minerals. Plus, when we buy fruits and veggies from a conventional supermarket, we have no idea how long it's been since they were picked. They're often flown in from the other side of the world, have been sitting in cold storage, and then had chemicals added to them before they hit our shelves, to speed up the ripening process and make them look presentable. Conventional tomatoes, for example, are picked green and then gassed to promote ripening, before hitting the supermarket shelves. Ever wondered why supermarket apples are so much shinier than organic apples? Many of them are actually coated in a toxic wax to give them this appeal.

Even with all of this information, conventional produce companies still have the hide to come out saying that organic produce is no more nutritious than their chemical-laden crops. How on Earth can that be? I don't know about you, but I would rather my food came without a coating of carcinogens.

There's also the argument that we can't be sure that what we're buying is actually organic. All you need to do is check that what you're buying has been 'certified organic' and you can be sure it complies with all the strict organic food quality regulations.

If cost is the subject of your protest, I have a rebuttal for that one too. It's all about priorities. Many of us are more than happy to spend money on gadgets, clothes, movies, restaurants, takeaway food and, dare I say it, doctor's visits and prescription medicines, but we don't like the idea of spending money on the best quality food. This is backward thinking. If you eat right, you will feel so good that you won't need to go to the doctor, you won't need as many of these superficial distractions, and you will look good in any clothes!

I actually don't think that organic produce is too expensive—it's just that conventional food is too cheap! I don't look at the price of conventional food anymore, because I don't deem it worthy enough to put in my body. So there's so point torturing myself over the fact that it would save me a few bucks!

However, if you're not quite ready to go 100% organic, start small and gradually make the transition. A good way to do this is by looking at the *Clean 15 vs The Dirty Dozen* list. Each year the wonderful people at the *Environmental Working Group* publish a list, indicating which conventional produce is the most contaminated by pesticides, and which is the cleanest.

The list is awesome for helping us determine which fruits and vegetables have the most pesticide residues and are the most essential to buy organic. You can lower your pesticide intake substantially by avoiding the 12 most contaminated fruits and vegetables and eating the least contaminated produce.

∞ EWG'S 2012 SHOPPER'S GUIDE TO PESTICIDES IN PRODUCE

Dirty Dozen Plus (buy these organic)

1. apples
2. celery
3. sweet bell peppers (capsicums)
4. peaches
5. strawberries
6. nectarines (imported)
7. grapes
8. spinach
9. lettuce
10. cucumbers
11. blueberries
12. potatoes

Plus (may contain pesticide residues of special concern)

+ green beans
+ kale/greens

Clean 15 (lowest in pesticide)

1. onions
2. sweet corn
3. pineapples
4. avocadoes
5. cabbages
6. sweet peas
7. asparagus
8. mangoes
9. eggplant
10. kiwi fruit

11. cantaloupes
12. sweet potatoes
13. grapefruit
14. watermelons
15. mushrooms

Note: Take this list with you when you go shopping.

If you do buy conventional produce, you can reduce the amount of pesticides by peeling the skins off or soaking for about 30-60 minutes in a sink filled with water and ¾ cup of apple cider vinegar. This will wash away some of the pesticides on the surface of the produce, but it still won't help with the toxic load that has soaked in through the skin. It also won't make up for the missing minerals, caused by the produce being grown in depleted soil.

∾ LOCAL YOKEL

While we're on the topic of the quality of our fruits and veggies, I want to mention the importance of buying local where possible. When you buy produce that comes from a farm close to you, you're not only supporting local business and reducing the environmental impact of transport, you're also ensuring that your food contains the highest amounts of nutrients possible. Fruits and veggies begin to lose their nutrients the moment they're picked from their source; so when you're buying food that has had to travel hundreds of miles to get to your plate, you're buying food that isn't fulfilling its potential. Buy local and you'll know that your food didn't have to travel too far to get to you, and most of its goodness will still be intact.

∞ RAW FOOD VERSUS COOKED FOOD

While we're on the topic of eating food as close to its natural state as possible, I have to explain why including raw food in the diet is important. I'm not into 100% raw diets—I don't like to gnaw on raw potatoes and grains—but there's something to be said about loading your plate up with raw food.

When we cook our food, especially at high heat, much of the enzymes, vitamins and minerals are lost. The all-important detoxifier, vitamin C, is destroyed once any heat is introduced. Kimberly Snyder, nutritionist and author of *The Beauty Detox Solution,* says that when we are young our bodies are populated by enzymes. As we age, we lose these enzymes, along with our youthful looks and energy. By eating a diet that is naturally packed with enzymes, we can replenish our lost supply.

∞ WHOLE LOTTA LOVE FOR WHOLE GRAINS

I know people who would rather eat their shoelaces than sit down to a bowl of rice or pasta. Not because they don't like the taste, but because they're so frightened by what they believe carbs will do to their ass. This fear is completely unjustified, if you select the right kind of carbohydrates to dine on.

We've already talked about why refined grains are damaging to our health, so now let's look at the flip side. **Whole grains** are a wonderful addition to your diet. They contain essential enzymes, iron, dietary fibre, vitamin E and B-complex vitamins. Because the body absorbs whole grains slowly, they provide sustained and high-quality energy. They also keep us feeling fuller for longer, and will help veggie food go a lot further.

When you choose organic whole grains, you can enjoy foods like rice, pasta and bread, without the guilt that usually creeps in after a refined grain blow-out. Whole grains have a completely different effect on our system. Because all of the parts of the grain are intact, our bodies know what to do with them. We absorb all of the nutrients that the grain carries. Whole grains are high in fibre, which means that the carbohydrates are absorbed much more slowly into our system. They don't raise our blood sugar and they help our digestive system run smoothly.

Great grains include …

∞ Brown rice

Brown rice contains the highest level of B vitamins out of all grains. It also contains iron, vitamin E, amino acids and linoleic acid. It takes longer to digest so provides us with prolonged energy. Brown rice must be soaked for at least eight hours before cooking, to deactivate its naturally occurring enzyme inhibitors.

∞ Quinoa

Pronounced 'keen-wah', quinoa has the highest nutritional profile and cooks the fastest of all grains. It is extremely high in protein and provides us with a lot of energy. Quinoa can take the place of rice; it only needs to be rinsed instead of soaked, and it only takes about 20 minutes to cook, compared to 40-45 minutes for brown rice.

Rye

Rye is very nutrient dense, supplying high levels of iron, calcium, potassium and zinc, as well as vitamin E and a variety of B vitamins. It's also a good source of protein and soluble fibre. Soluble fibre helps us to feel fuller longer, as it slows down the breakdown of carbohydrates and sugars. Rye flour has far lower gluten content than wheat, and is excellent for use with a sourdough starter.

Spelt

Spelt is known as ancient wheat, but it doesn't cause the same allergic reactions or intolerances as wheat. It's high in fibre and manganese and contains good amounts of copper, niacin and protein.

Buckwheat

Also known as kasha, buckwheat is actually a fruit seed related to rhubarb. Although buckwheat has the look, feel, taste and versatility of grain, buckwheat is not technically grain, and it contains no gluten. It contains all of the essential amino acids, making it one of the few vegetarian sources of complete protein to equal the protein of fish or meat in quality. Buckwheat has a nutty, rich flavour that complements many dishes.

Millet

With a similar consistency to couscous, millet makes a great wheat-free substitute for dishes that call for this small, round grain.

Whichever grain product you choose, always be sure to read the ingredients label. Choose an organic brand and make sure that the product doesn't contain any preservatives or additives. You can usually pick up breads and pastas that list olive oil and sea salt as the last ingredients—these ones are good choices.

— WHAT'S THE GO WITH GLUTEN?

Giving your body a break from gluten can be a great help when it comes to losing weight, clearing up skin conditions and health issues and promoting an overall feeling of wellness. Integrative doctor, Dr Frank Lipman, says that, even if you don't have an allergy or sensitivity to gluten (both of which are very common these days), gluten can impose a burden on your digestive system. Gluten is a hard-to-digest protein that can be irritating and exhausting to your system. It generally requires a lot of work on your body's behalf to be broken down. Therefore, by removing gluten from the diet, your body is free to work on healing other issues. The liver, digestive system and immune system are given time to recover.

Gluten can be found in grains such as wheat, barley, rye, bulgur, couscous, farina, kamut, kasha, semolina, spelt and triticale. Choose gluten-free alternatives, like brown rice pasta instead of regular pasta, basmati rice, brown rice, buckwheat, millet and quinoa.

Oats are generally considered a gluten grain, however they don't naturally contain it. Oats do not contain the 'gliadin' protein that people have a hard time digesting and breaking down. The problem is that cross-contamination occurs, when oats are produced using the same machinery and equipment as other gluten-containing products. Look for 'gluten-free' oats, to be sure you're consuming the pure stuff.

∞ LOVELY LEGUMES

Before my cancer diagnosis, I was a massive meat eater. I ate it at least twice a day, and didn't feel full and satisfied without it. When I became a plant eater, there was one little dietary element that saved me from feeling starved: **the legume.** These days, I'm more than satisfied with my plant-based diet, but in the beginning legumes were a transitioning-phase lifesaver.

Adding legumes (think lentils, chickpeas, beans, etcetera etcetera) is the best way to add a hearty, filling component to a plant-based meal. They're packed with protein, fibre, vitamins, minerals and phytochemicals. They are economical, filling, and go a long way when it comes to stretching out a meal.

Here's a list of legumes to try ...

Chickpeas

Tasting like a cross between a pea and a nut, chickpeas are my favourite form of legume. But they have to be the fresh ones. If you've only tasted tinned chickpeas, the fresh ones are going to blow your mind. Soak them overnight or for eight hours, then add them straight to salads and wraps, cook them in curries, soups and stir fries, or blend them up to make hummus. Another trick I've recently discovered is to bake the soaked chickpeas for about 30-40 minutes. They come out of the oven tasting like peanuts! And when you whiz them in a blender, they taste like peanut butter!

Cooking time: 120-180 minutes

Lentils

Small, flat and disk-shaped, lentils are a good source of vitamin B, fibre, iron, protein and phosphorus, which is an essential mineral that every cell in the body requires for normal function. Choose from red, brown, yellow and French varieties. Lentils are awesome in curries, stews, soups, dips and salads.

Cooking time: 30-45 minutes.

Snap peas

Also known as shelling peas, snap peas have plump pods with a bright green colour and crisp texture. They are a good source of vitamins and minerals including vitamin A, vitamin B6, vitamin C, vitamin K, iron, potassium, magnesium and riboflavin. I love eating these peas raw, straight from the pod, but they can also be cooked to bring out a sweeter flavour.

Beans

Beans are a form of legume. Azuki beans are predominantly used in Japanese dishes; black beans and kidney beans are great if you're cooking Mexican; and fresh sprouted mung beans are fantastic in salads. You can also choose from lima beans, fava beans, pinto beans, navy beans and cannellini beans.

Cooking times:

      Azuki 45-60 minutes
      Black (turtle) 60-90 minutes
      Cannellini 90-120 minutes
      Fava 60-90 minutes
      Kidney 60-90 minutes
      Lima beans 60-90 minutes
      Navy 60-90 minutes
      Pinto 90 minutes

∞ HOW TO INCREASE DIGESTIBILITY AND REDUCE BLOATINESS

Love legumes, but hate how farty and bloaty they make you? Don't we all! Good news is that there are certain steps you can take to make legumes easier on your digestive system, to eliminate these embarrassing and uncomfortable side effects:

∞ Soak legumes for a couple of hours before cooking them.

∞ Use a pressure cooker. This also cuts down on cooking time.

∞ Chew thoroughly.

∞ Try red lentils instead of brown, as they are easier on your system.

∞ Watch what you are eating your legumes with. They combine best with greens or non-starchy vegetables and seaweeds.

∞ Add fennel or cumin near the end of cooking, to help prevent gas.

- Add kombu or kelp seaweed to improve flavour and digestion, add minerals and nutrients, and speed up the cooking process.

- Pour a little apple cider vinegar into the water in the last stages of cooking. This softens the legumes and breaks down protein chains and indigestible compounds.

- Take digestive enzymes with your meal.

Note: Avoid giving legumes to children under 18 months, as they haven't developed the gastric enzymes to digest them properly.

— IS SOY A GOOD SUBSTITUTE?

The short answer to this question is 'no'. Nothing makes me cringe quite so much as seeing well-meaning health seekers swapping meat for fake meats, dairy for soy milk and adding tofu to everything.

Many experts claim that soy is good for everyone. 'It helps get you through menopause!' 'It helps prevent breast cancer!' 'It is the ideal alternative to dairy!' Then there are the studies that show that soy is downright evil, suppressing thyroid function, messing with our hormones and acting as a potent carcinogenic.

So, who are we to believe? Honestly, it's really hard to say, but my motto with this kind of thing is, *If in doubt, leave it out.* In my opinion, there's just too much information pointing to the detrimental effects of soy to eat it freely. Plus, even those who claim that soy does have some benefits will agree that most of it is heavily processed and often genetically modified so should only be consumed in moderation. What is moderation though? I don't want to be putting even moderate amounts of toxins into my body. Plus, soy is found in almost everything—from baby formula and burgers to all processed foods. If you eat processed foods, you literally can't get away from it. It doesn't even have to be stated on the ingredients label!

Hundreds of epidemiological, clinical and laboratory studies link soy to malnutrition, digestive distress, thyroid dysfunction, cognitive decline, reproductive disorders, infertility, birth defects, immune system breakdown, heart disease and cancer. If you want to research soy more and make up your own mind about this food, I recommend you pick up a copy of *The Whole Soy Story* by Kaayla T Daniel PhD or read Elaine Hollingsworth's thoughts in her book, *Take Control of Your Health and Escape the Sickness Industry.*

The only time soy is okay to eat is if it's fermented (in the form of tempeh or miso), but this should still be kept to a minimal portion of the diet. This is because fermentation releases nutrients and transforms soybeans into a nutritious food.

∞ THE DEAL WITH SUPPLEMENTS

I'm the first to admit that taking supplements is a pain in the butt. It can be expensive, it's a bit of an inconvenience, and I would much prefer to receive all of the nutrients I need from food. However, the reality is that our food these days just doesn't cut it—even if you eat a clean, organic diet. We need supplements to make up for the areas our bodies are lacking in.

We need these additional nutrients because our soils, our farming techniques, our food processing and our food distribution system result in nutrient depleted foods, says Dr Mark Hyman. *Even with the perfect diet, the combination of our depleted soils, the storage and transportation of our foods around the world, the genetic alterations of traditional heirloom species, and the increased stress and nutritional demand resulting from a toxic environment make it almost impossible for us to get the vitamins and minerals we need just from the foods we eat. The evidence shows that we can't get away from the need for nutritional supplements.*

Everyone's supplement needs are different, so I highly recommend being tested by a naturopath or an integrative doctor, to find out what your body specifically needs. Taking targeted supplements will save you money, and you won't be putting anything into your body that you don't need.

Another reason I recommend working with an expert on your supplement plan is so they can prescribe the best quality vitamins and minerals. Purchasing them from any old pharmacy or health food store won't guarantee that you'll be consuming something of quality. In fact, more often than not, store-bought supplements are made up of mostly synthetic ingredients, which can do more harm than good.

As I've said, our bodies are not designed to consume synthetics and this applies to supplements as well. It confuses them. Instead of nourishing us, synthetic ingredients rob us of nutrients, because our bodies mine minerals from their own reserves to make up for what's missing in the pill or food or whatever we've consumed. Our bodies know what to do with ingredients that are whole and genuinely natural and they will take as much as they need while excreting the rest. When the ingredient is synthetic, the excess is stored in our cells and fatty tissues and leads to toxicity.

Just because something claims to be natural, it doesn't mean that it is. In a similar form of sorcery to the beauty industry, vitamins can be labelled as natural if they contain as little as 10% of the natural form of the vitamin. So, that 'natural' vitamin you're consuming may actually be made up of 90% synthetic chemicals. The *Organic Consumers Association* recommends looking for products that contain '100 percent plant-based' or '100 percent animal-based' on the product's label.

What to look for on the label

1. The food source: A food source will indicate that the product has been made from something natural. A missing food source indicates it was made in a test tube. Look for food sources such as yeast, fish, vegetable and citrus. Also, identify whole foods in the ingredient list, instead of the particular nutrient.
2. Salt forms: Salt forms (like acetate, bitartrate, chloride, gluconate, hydrochloride, nitrate and succinate) are synthetic ingredients added to supplements to increase the stability of the vitamin or mineral.
3. These keywords: Words that end in 'ide' or 'ate' (like chloride, hydrochloride, acetate or nitrate) indicate that the product contains salt forms, which are synthetics. If you see the letters 'dl' before the name of an ingredient, this tells you it's synthetic.

Common synthetic vitamins to avoid

Look for clues on your vitamin's label that offer insight into the origin of the vitamin:

Vitamin A: acetate and palmitate
Vitamin B1 (thiamine): thiamine mononitrate, thiamine hydrochloride
Vitamin B2 (riboflavin): riboflavin
Pantothenic acid: calcium d-pantothenate
Vitamin B6 (pyridoxine): pyridoxine hydrochloride
Vitamin B12: cobalamin
PABA (para-aminobenzoic acid): aminobenzoic acid
Folic acid: pteroylglutamic acid
Choline: choline chloride, choline bitartrate
Biotin: d-biotin
Vitamin C (ascorbic acid): ascorbic acid
Vitamin D: irradiated ergosteral, calciferol
Vitamin E: dl-alpha tocopherol, dl-alpha tocopherol acetate or succinate

Note: The 'dl' form of any vitamin is synthetic.

Other toxic ingredients to avoid in supplements

Magnesium stearate (or stearic acid)
Monosodium glutamate (MSG) disguised as 'natural flavours'
Carnauba wax is used in car wax and shoe polish
Titanium dioxide is a carcinogen

Again, I highly recommend you consult a naturopath or integrative doctor, to work out the best supplement plan for you. This is the best way to not only make sure you're only taking what you need, but they will be able to prescribe reputable brands. Still, grill them about the ingredients and make it very clear that you will only consume something if it's 100% natural and 0% synthetic.

Supplements I recommend

∞ A good probiotic

Look for bacteria that give off lactic acid as a by-product of their metabolism. Look for strains like bifidobacteria, boulardii, acidophilus and lactobacillus. Make sure it is high in lactobacillus and bifidobacterium—the count should be in the billions. You should also look for capsules that are vegetarian and come enteric-coated. This coating keeps the bacteria safely inside, until the capsule makes its way to your small intestine.

∞ Digestive enzymes

When you switch to an all-plant and mostly raw diet, you can often experience a lot of gas, bloating and digestive discomfort. Digestive enzymes assist in the digestion of foods and help to eliminate these issues.

∞ Niacin (vitamin B3)

Niacin ruptures the fat cells that store toxins, releasing those stored toxins to be eliminated. It also assists in the digestion of protein, lowers cholesterol and helps to open capillary circulation and bring freshly-oxygenated blood to all the body tissues. There are two types of niacin—nicotinic acid and nicotinamide. Nicotinic acid is the correct one to take. Nicotinamide (also known as niacinamide) can be potentially toxic to the liver. Always buy the active form, not the slow release form, and be sure to buy the niacin that gives you the niacin flush.

∞ Milk thistle

This herb has awesome detoxifying and liver protective qualities and can protect against some severe liver toxins.

∞ B12

We don't get B12 from plant sources, so a supplement is needed for all vegetarians and vegans. Always use the methylcobalamin form of B12 and not the cheaper, synthetic (and more common) cyanocobalamin.

∞ FERMENTED FOODS

Probiotic and digestive enzyme supplements are extremely helpful, but we shouldn't overlook the benefits of including fermented foods in the diet. Fermented foods are a staple in diets around the world, but for some sad reason the western world neglects them and their digestive powers. We're more inclined to pop laxative pills and powders instead, **after** we get all clogged up. Fermented foods, as in raw, cultured vegetables, are Mother Nature's answer to aiding our digestion. They replenish our supply of friendly bacteria in the gut. And when the gut is happy, so is the rest of our body. When the gut's good bacteria colonies are thriving, we're able to digest our food and absorb the nutrients. We lose weight, skin conditions clear up, cravings subside and many unexplained health issues may dissipate.

You can buy fermented foods and drinks like kimchi, sauerkraut, kombucha and kefir from the fridge section of your organic store. However, you can also make your own quite easily. There are a tonne of recipes online. When you make your own, you can also control the amount of salt you include.

ARE YOU FULL OF SHIT?

CHAPTER FIVE

∞ It's all well and good to be concerned with what you're putting into your body, but perhaps of even more importance is what is coming out of it. Yes, I'm talking about poop. If your internal plumbing system is on the fritz, your health will be suffering, you'll hold onto excess weight, and it will also show up in your skin. Nasty, nasty, nasty. The late, great Dr Max Gerson is famous for saying, *Never let the sun set unless you have a bowel movement.* Smart man. To maintain optimum health, we need to keep things running smoothly on our internal freeway.

The digestive system includes the entire path that food and nutrients take on their journey through the body, from the mouth and oesophagus to the small and large intestines. It doesn't matter if you have the best diet or the worst, if your digestive system is not functioning properly it won't be able to deliver the required nutrition. Chronic fatigue, premature ageing, arthritis, poor skin and hair quality, toxicity, allergies, cancer and many other diseases can result. Foods that are not properly digested will ferment and putrefy in the intestinal tract and produce toxic by-products that are absorbed back into the body.

Poor digestion is generally caused by insufficient diet, dehydration, eating too fast, not chewing your food and stress. Eating a lot of refined, high-sugar foods, instead of fresh, fibre- and enzyme-rich fruits and vegetables, is likely to cause digestive problems. The same goes for eating meat that has been pumped with antibiotics.

— WHY STRESS SCREWS WITH DIGESTION

It's nothing new that stress ravages your health. It causes cortisol levels to rise, adds pressure to your adrenals, hinders your immune system, messes with your hormones and keeps your mind separated from your body. But the one health/stress association we hear little about is the fact that stress interferes with digestion. When we experience stressful situations, our bodies are unable to absorb any nutrients from our food. It doesn't matter how much good food you eat, if you live a highly-strung lifestyle, all of the brown rice and broccoli in the world won't do you much good.

Dr Nicholas Gonzalez says that the two branches of our autonomic nervous system play crucial roles in our healing process. He says that our sympathetic nervous system's job is to help our body deal with stress by diverting blood to the brain and the muscles. This is so that, in times of stress, we can think quickly and our muscles can react quickly. Sympathetic nerves divert energy away from the gut to the brain and muscles. While this is happening, our entire digestive system is shut down.

The parasympathetic system works in the opposite way, taking advantage of our restful state at night, when we are sleeping to repair and rebuild our bodies. The parasympathetic system is responsible for digestion. It increases the efficiency of digestion, secretion of hydrochloric acid, enzymes from the pancreas, and the bile salts from the liver. Dr Gonzales says that this system increases the absorption of nutrients, stimulates the repair of damaged tissues, and is basically a reparative system.

So what does this all mean? First of all, it's proof that the majority of our healing happens when we are sleeping, which is why it's so important to get enough quality sleep each night. It also means that, if you're constantly under stress, all of your energy will be diverted away from your gut. Your digestive system won't ever be given the chance to perform its super important task of absorbing life-giving nutrients from your food.

Tips for tiptop digestion

- Start your day by drinking lemon juice in warm water—this is great for your pipes, alkalising, cleansing, and a great way to gently wake up your system (much better than slapping your body awake with coffee).
- Sip on apple cider vinegar in warm water about half an hour before a meal. This can help to stimulate digestive juices and improve the breakdown of food.

~ Eat in a relaxed environment and take the time to enjoy your meals. Chew your food!

~ Improve your ability to cope with stress by regularly practising meditation and deep breathing.

~ Drink herbal teas such as peppermint, lemongrass and ginger, to provide relief from digestive discomfort.

~ Include cooked veggies in your diet. These guys are easier to digest and will help push the raw food through.

~ Eat light to heavy. If you drink a fresh juice or smoothie or eat fresh fruit, veggies or salad after a heavy meal that takes time to digest, the lighter stuff will sit on top of the slower, heavier stuff, and have time to ferment and acidify. Prevent this from happening by always eating the lighter portion of your meal first. My order goes like this: soup, salad, cooked veggies, brown rice.

~ Don't drink water while you eat. Consuming liquids with your food will dilute the gastric juices and hinder the digestion and absorption process.

~ Eat foods high in fibre, such as whole grains, organic vegetables, fruits and oats.

~ Always eat fruit on its own. Fruit digests the fastest, and can be in and out of your body in 30 minutes. But if you eat it with or after something that takes longer to digest, it will have to wait its turn and will sit in your system with time to ferment and create acidity.

- Swap processed, refined sugar and salt-laden food for organic, fresh fruits and vegetables.

- Source a quality probiotic supplement, to help put the good bacteria back into your body.

— ALL ABOUT ENEMAS

Now that we've covered the importance of digestion, we need to discuss elimination. I'm not shy about my affection for the coffee enema. While I usually talk about it in relation to its liver cleansing ability, I'm bringing it up now because it also helps you poop.

First of all, enemas and colonics are two very different things. However, many people get them confused and think they do the same job. Colonics are mechanically fed and use water to flush out your whole colon; while enemas just work the lower part of the colon and the liver. They are gentler, and can be self-administered in the comfort of your own bathroom. Coffee enemas are also irreplaceable when it comes to moving toxins out of your system. They stimulate the liver and increase bile production, to excrete toxins more rapidly. They have the amazing ability to rescue people from all kinds of ailments including headaches, hangovers, colds and flu. Coffee enemas were my greatest ally when healing my body from cancer. They continue to be a regular part of my daily routine.

I recommend coffee enemas to anyone embarking on a detox. When we clean up our diets and get stuck into juices and smoothies, we naturally stir up toxins that have building up in our bodies over the years. It's our liver's job to eliminate the toxins, but because we live in such a toxic world, they have their work cut out for them. This is where the coffee enema comes in, giving your liver a hand by relieving some of the work load.

Coffee enema 101 procedure

1. Buy yourself an enema kit. There are all kinds available, but I prefer buckets with a flat base so that you can sit them on a chair or your bathroom bench. Buckets come in both plastic and stainless steel. Look online and see what's available.

2. Use organic, medium ground, light/medium roast coffee. Boil enough coffee for two enemas just in case you can't hold the first one and want to try again. For two enemas, bring one litre of water to the boil in a pot on the stove.

3. Once boiling, remove from the stove and add six table-spoons of coffee. Turn stove down to low, then return the pot to the burner. Boil for three minutes, and then reduce to a simmer for another 15 minutes. Remove from the stove and strain the coffee, using a very fine mesh strainer or cheesecloth.

4. Add 8 ounces (250ml) of coffee to your bucket and top it up with 16 ounces (500ml) of purified water. Make sure the liquid is body temperature—you don't want it too cold, and you definitely don't want it too hot. I've been there and it's not nice. Plus, once the coffee is on its way into your bottom, it's too late to do anything about it.

MAKE PEACE WITH YOUR PLATE

5. Lay a yoga mat and/or towels on your bathroom floor (for padding). Cover the part of the towel where your bottom will sit with a disposable white paper pad (ours have blue plastic backs and we buy them from the pharmacy). This will catch any mess and save you from having to wash so many towels!

6. Release the clasp on the tube and let the liquid run through the tube and drip a bit into the sink. This will remove any air bubbles.

7. Hang or sit the enema bucket on a chair or sit it on the bathroom counter. It needs to be higher than you, so that gravity can do its thing. You won't want it too high for your first few enemas, as you may have trouble retaining the liquid.

8. Lie on your right side with your legs pulled up towards your chest. Lube up the end of the tube with a bit of coconut oil and insert about two inches into your bottom.

9. Let the solution flow all the way in and tighten the clamp before removing it. Then lie back and relax for 15 minutes (or as long as you can). I like to read a book or watch something on my laptop to pass the time.

10. When the time is up, get up off the floor, sit on the toilet and release all of the coffee and toxins into the loo.

If you're planning on doing regular coffee enemas, it's important to replenish your body's electrolyte levels with fresh juices, coconut water, fresh salads and vegetables. The amount you do is totally up to you. On Gerson Therapy, the general rule is one coffee enema for every four juices.

You could start with one a week, one every couple of days, or however many you are comfortable with.

Want to see a coffee enema in action? For a PG demonstration, go to: thewellnesswarrior.com.au/2012/10/ healthtalks-episode-2-all-about-coffee-enemas/

∞ COLONICS

Colonic hydrotherapy is another great addition to your cleansing regime, as it will get into your colon and help to clear out any gunk and sludge that has been holed up in there. Unlike enemas, you can't give yourself a colonic and it's important that you find a reputable therapist to administer it for you. Gravity fed colonics are generally the best way to go. They are gentler than the hydraulic kind and, if the therapist knows what they are doing, the process should be relatively comfortable.

Adverse opinions against colonics claim that they strip the colon of good bacteria as well as bad, so it's important to replenish your supply by taking probiotic supplements and eating fermented, probiotic-rich foods.

Having major issues pooping?
If you're constipated to the point of frustration, I have a sure-fire solution for you. It may make you screw up your nose and gag with resistance, but I'm tellin' you it'll work a treat. I recently tested this out on a friend of mine who hadn't been to the toilet for a number two in just under a week. She was desperate. So, I went over to her house with a bottle of castor oil and instructions on how to administer

the castor oil treatment we were taught at the Gerson clinic. It's this easy:

1. Take two tablespoons of castor oil orally.
2. Immediately chase with a cup of black coffee sweetened with a teaspoon of raw sugar. (This stimulates things and helps to push the castor oil through)
3. Wait for the magic to happen.

This procedure may make you feel a bit sick in the guts and lethargic (it always made me feel hungover), but that just means it's working. Before you know it, the castor oil will have made its way through your digestive system, unblocking any blockages, sweeping up any debris, and activating poopage. It's best taken first thing in the morning on an empty stomach, and be sure you're able to stay close to a toilet during the hours after taking it.

HEALTHY ALTERNATIVES TO YOUR NASTY OLD HABITS

Healthy eating rocks my socks off. But if it weren't for the fact that eating this way can also be amazingly tasty, I doubt that I would have the same devotion to it as I do. The thing is, being healthy is not as horrible on your taste buds as many people believe. You just need to be creative, garner some imagination, and learn all about the ways you can swap your old nasty habits for super healthy alternatives that are just as tasty. Here are some suggestions you might like.

∞ SUGAR
You don't have to give up sugar altogether (cue happy dance). You just need to source a natural sweetener that suits you. Good news is that there are plenty of them. You're welcome!

Raw honey

Unless you're a strict vegan, I would say that raw honey is the sweetener of choice. It's definitely my favourite. Raw honey (which has not been pasteurised or filtered, and ideally taken directly from the hive) is a treasure chest of nutritional value and medicinal remedies. It contains an abundance of vitamins and minerals and is a natural, powerful medicine, both internally and externally. Superfoods expert David Wolfe says to look for wild honey, because it is lower in free fructose and higher in trace mineral content.

Maple syrup

Maple syrup is my favourite sweetener for baking and making raw vegan desserts. It's also full of super beneficial minerals. However, be sure to buy authentic organic maple syrup. The conventional stuff is usually fake-coloured sugar water and not at all healthy.

Dates (or date paste)

Dates are very sweet, but they are great because they are packed with fibre. If using whole dates, fresh Medjool dates are the best. If paste is required, buy organic date paste or make your own by blending or cooking dates with a little water over low heat.

Stevia

If you're diabetic, suffer from candida or cancer, or you're worried about your blood sugar levels, stevia is the way to go. It won't mess with your blood sugar levels at all. The green leaves are better than the white extract though. It's super sweet, so you only need a small amount.

∞ Yacon

Yacon (a relative to the Jerusalem artichoke) is commonly available as dehydrated chips and as a syrup. The syrup is rich in iron and only mildly glycemic. Just be sure to buy certified organic.

∞ Coconut sugar

With a minimal effect on blood sugar levels, coconut sugar is emerging as a favourite among vegans and raw foodies. It isn't technically raw though, being the boiled down sap harvested from unopened coconut blossoms. I love it if I want to add sweetness to an Asian-flavoured dish.

∞ Coconut nectar

This is the syrup version of coconut sugar. It's an awesome choice for a subtle sweet flavour in desserts.

∞ Molasses

If you can handle its rich flavour, molasses is a super healthy addition to your diet. It's rich in vitamins and minerals, but be sure to select unsulfured, organic sugarcane molasses.

∞ FAT

Contrary to pretty much all health marketing from the last few decades, fat does not make us fat. One of the biggest mistakes the food industry made was to label fat as bad. We need fat. Certain fats are essential to our daily diet and for the health of our central nervous system. For instance, did you know that our brains are 60 per cent fat? The best thing you can do for yourself is stop scouring supermarket shelves for the words 'low fat'.

Here are some of my favourite fat sources ...

∞ Coconut oil

My gosh, I love me some coconut oil! This saturated fat has received a bad rap for yonks, but finally people are starting to wise up to its many benefits. It's healthy to cook with, it aids in weight loss, it won't mess with cholesterol, and you can also use it topically to prevent wrinkles. Our bodies actually need a certain amount of saturated fat, and when it comes from the coconut it has the added benefit of not raising your cholesterol.

∞ Avocado

Avocados are great for heart health, they lower cholesterol, are an excellent source of glutathione (the master detoxifier), and are also super high in vitamin E.

∞ Nuts

Nuts are awesome. Not only are they great for your heart, but they are also really satiating and a good source of protein.

- ∞ **Walnuts** are a good source of protein, fibre and magnesium. They have a high level of alpha-linolenic acid, a type of brain-boosting omega-3 fatty acid.

- ∞ **Brazil nuts** are high in selenium, which is super important for your thyroid.

- **Almonds** are high in fibre and calcium, and are an excellent source of vitamin E.

- **Cashews** give you nearly 10% of your daily requirement of iron in a single serving. They are a good source of folate and vitamin K, which helps keep bones strong and blood clotting normally.

- **Pistachios** are rich in lutein, an antioxidant that's also found in leafy greens and is important for healthy vision and skin; plus one serving gives you almost as much potassium as a small banana.

- **Macadamia nuts** are high in fibre and protein, and rich in vital minerals like potassium, manganese, calcium, iron, magnesium and zinc.

∞ Flaxseed oil

Flaxseed oil is one of the best plant-based sources of omega-3 and omega-6 essential fatty acids. I love it as a salad dressing.

∞ Butter

Unless you're vegan, organic grass-fed butter is a great choice. It contains a number of natural fatty acids that are excellent for the body. Butter is an excellent source of fat-soluble vitamins, such as vitamin A, D, E and K.

∞ ESSENTIAL FATTY ACIDS

Essential fatty acids, or EFAs, are fatty acids that are crucial for our health, but that our bodies cannot synthesise. Hence, why they are essential.

˙˙˙˙˙ Omega-3s

Powerful and essential fatty acids, found in foods like fish, flaxseed, hemp seed, chia seed and walnuts. Omega-3 fatty acids are essential elements for the brain and the nervous system. Omega-3 is great for warding off cancer, heart disease and even Alzheimer's.

˙˙˙˙˙ Omega-6

An essential fatty acid that is critical for your health but, unlike omega-3, too much of omega-6 is not a good thing. Too much omega-6 can overpower and cancel out the benefits of omega-3. Maintaining the right balance between these two omegas is vital for your health. Omega-6 is found in egg yolk and most plant oils like corn, peanut, poppy seed, safflower, canola, sesame, soy and sunflower.

˙˙˙˙˙ WHICH OIL IS BEST TO COOK WITH?

Not all oils are suitable for cooking. There are only a few that are stable enough to handle the heat. The ones that aren't will become rancid on heating, causing inflammation in the body—and inflammation is the root cause of pretty much all disease.

- ˙˙˙˙˙ **Heat stable** oils (can stand high heat): coconut, butter, ghee, macadamia

- ˙˙˙˙˙ **Moderately stable** oils (can stand moderate heat): sesame, peanut, hazelnut, almond, olive

- ˙˙˙˙˙ **Unstable** oils (never, ever heat): sunflower, corn, flaxseed

∞ CHOCOLATE

The day I discovered that chocolate is actually a superfood was the day I pledged my eternal love for Mother Nature. She sure did well with that one.

Chocolate is made of cocoa, which is derived from cacao. Raw organic cacao (pronounced cuh-cow) is extremely healthy and ridiculously high in antioxidants, magnesium and vitamin C. This only applies to chocolate in its raw, whole, natural state though.

Most of the chocolate you see at the supermarket has had all the goodness processed, cooked and refined out of it. What you're left with is a bar of mostly sugar, milk fat, hydrogenated oils and artificial flavourings. Studies have shown that dairy products actually block the absorption of antioxidants in chocolate.

The cacao that is used to make mass-produced chocolate is generally sourced cheaply from countries like Africa, where they have the nasty Capra beetle. When this cacao arrives in Australia, quarantine treats it aggressively with methylbromide gas fumigation and irradiation, to kill any remnants of the insects. Sounds delicious, right? And that's just the beginning of the nutrient-depleting, chemical-adding process of turning cacao into the mass-produced, profit-rendering chocolate we often treat ourselves to.

∞ DAIRY

Dairy may not be all it's cracked up to be. But the good news is that there are plenty of healthy ways to recreate the creamy consistency it provides to many comfort foods. For instance, did you know that you can make cheesecake out of cashews and that it actually tastes way better than the moo-juice derived kind? Whoever discovered that nifty trick deserves a trophy. Cashews can also be used to make cream and sour cream. Milk can be made from oats, rice or pretty much any nut or seed; ice cream can be made from coconut or nuts; and yoghurt can be made from coconut cream.

You'll find recipes for all of these in Chapter 8.

Some more considerations:

∞ BREAD

Ditch white bread and the stuff that comes with a textbook-long ingredients list. Swap it for organic bread made from whole grains. Choose from breads made from rye, spelt or oat flour, and just make sure that the ingredients are minimal and all natural and organic.

∞ PASTA

There are plenty of great pasta alternatives on the market these days. I love quinoa pasta, mung bean pasta, brown rice pasta, black bean pasta or kelp noodles. You can also make pasta from zucchini, by using a vegetable spiralling tool.

∞ SALAD DRESSING

Forget the bottled stuff. It's full of sugar and preservatives, plus it's so easy to whip up your own. I love using flaxseed oil and raw apple cider vinegar on my salad. You can also get creative by mixing these two together and adding something fun like honey, mustard, ginger and herbs. If you want it creamy, add nuts or seeds.

∞ FLAVOURINGS

Instead of using bottles and jars of sauces to flavour your food, use potent and natural herbs and spices. Try curry powder, cumin, turmeric, cayenne pepper, chilli, basil, oregano, dill, rosemary, sage, thyme, coriander, lemon juice and lime juice.

∞ BREAKFAST CEREAL

Some packaged breakfast cereals should be considered junk food—they are so full of sugar, preservatives and additives. They should definitely not be considered a healthy start to the day. Instead, make up your own cereal out of rolled oats (toasted if you like), goji berries, nuts, seeds, coconut etc. Just add homemade nut milk.

∞ PIZZA

Make your own homemade pizza by using an organic whole grain base, like spelt or rye. Then add organic tomato paste, and layer on the veggies of your choice. Add cashew cheese, brazil nut parmesan or goat fetta (if you're not vegan) to the top.

EXPERT WORD ▌ CYNDI O'MEARA

We seem to be cutting everything out of our diet. It was first salt, then fat, and now it's sugar. I don't necessarily think we should be cutting those foods out. I actually think they're very important in our diet, but it's about quality not quantity. When you look at the different salts and the different fats and the different sugars is when you look at what's best for the human body and what the body has biologically evolutionarily grown up to eat over the last million years. We ate salt, fat and sugar throughout our evolution. The whole sugars—the sugars that have still got vitamins, minerals and nutrients and are in their whole form—are the ones we should be eating. Where as the sugars that we should be cutting out are the refined sugars and the artificial sweeteners. My rule of thumb is that if it's made or processed by man, keep away from it. If it's from nature, go for it and enjoy it, but have a balance as well.

Cyndi O'Meara is one of Australia's leading, most unapologetic and provocative nutritionists, blazing a trail with her message that, when it comes to food, Mother Nature always knows best. She is an international speaker, a TV and radio presenter, and the author of the best selling book, *Changing Habits Changing Lives.*

Putting All This Into Practice

CHAPTER SEVEN

∞ I hope that by this stage in the book you're feeling super inspired and excited about implementing everything we've just chewed over in your own life. Up until now, we've been in the 'theory' section of your newfound relationship with food. Now it's time to get stuck into the 'practice' portion.

Feeling overwhelmed? That's to be expected. You've just absorbed a heap of information that has probably challenged you, opened your mind, and maybe even pissed you off a little. Don't worry—I've been there. When I was first researching all of this stuff, I would get so angry every time I read about one of my favourite foods being 'bad' for me. I was almost tempted to put my head back in the sand and bask in the comfort of my ignorance. But once you learn all of this stuff, it's impossible to 'unlearn' it, and it's definitely impossible to ignore it.

So, if you're ready to continue along this path, I want to impart all of the wisdom I possibly can to make sure the rest of the journey is as smooth and enjoyable as it can be. It's one thing to digest the information, but the life-transforming power comes from putting it into practice. You will never truly know just how amazing this lifestyle is until you live it firsthand.

In this chapter, I'm going to give you some tips and tricks for getting started and for making peace with your plate in the real world. We're going to cover everything from making food fun at home, to making it easy to be healthy while you're out and about—even while you're travelling.

I don't mean to toot my own horn here, but I genuinely walk my talk when it comes to this stuff. I'm not just sitting on my soapbox spewing information: I practise what I'm preaching. In all of the years since I started on this journey, I've not strayed once. In the beginning it was tough, and I would be forever bugging my friends for sniffs of their hot chips or burgers. But these days, I can honestly say that I wouldn't change anything about the way I eat. I've stopped saying 'I can't eat that' when presented with something that will put my health into a decline, and have started saying, 'Thanks, but I choose not to eat that.' It's no longer a chore—it's a choice. I actually have a lot of fun getting creative with this lifestyle and making it work for me.

Now, without further adieu, let's get into some tools and advice for maintaining a peaceful relationship with food outside of these pages.

⚬⚬⚬ GETTING YOUR KITCHEN READY

Life will be a whole lot more peaceful if you invest in some quality kitchen equipment. You don't need to break the bank, but believe me when I say that you will save money in the long run, if you prioritise kitchen gadgets and buy the best equipment you can afford. Here are five must-have items:

1. **A blender**

   A good blender is an absolute must-have for making smoothies, nut milks, desserts and sauces. Flip back to Chapter 4 to suss out the right blender for you.

2. **A juicer**

   You will need a juicer to make juices. No, you cannot just use your blender. A blender won't remove the fibre, which is what we want when making juice. A run-down on juicers can be found back in Chapter 4.

3. **A veggie spiralling tool**

   If you want to make sexy spaghetti out of zucchini and noodles out of carrots, you need to buy yourself a vegetable spiralling tool. A veggie peeler will do a similar job, but not quite. These tools also go by the name of a 'spiraliser' or a *Spirooli*. A good kitchen store should stock these. If not, just google.

4. **A nut milk bag**

   Since I've convinced you to swap moo juice for nut sauce (I know, that's gross), you're going to be chomping at the bit to make some from scratch. It's easy and fun. You can use an old stocking or thin cloth, but a nut milk bag will make the process even easier. Ask for one at your local organic store, or have a look online.

5. **Non-toxic cookware**

Non-stick pans are a great idea in theory. They allow us to cook whatever we want without oil, without sticking, without any mess. Genius! Until we realise that teflon and other non-stick substances are highly toxic. According to tests commissioned by the *Environmental Working Group* (EWG), in the two to five minutes that cookware coated with teflon is heating on a conventional stove top, temperatures can exceed the point where the coating breaks apart and emits toxic particles and gases. At various temperatures, these coatings can release at least six toxic gases, including two carcinogens.

When pans with these coatings get scratched during cooking, small amounts of plastic and leached aluminum cling to the food and are then ingested by us. A 2005 study by the EWA, in collaboration with Commonwealth, found perflourooctanoic acid (PFOA), a chemical found in such pans and a known carcinogen, in the umbilical cord blood of newborns. *John Hopkins Medical Center* did a similar test in 2006, where PFOA was found to be present in the umbilical cord blood of 99% of the 300 infants tested.

What should we cook with?

Do not use:

∞ aluminium
∞ teflon
∞ copper
∞ lead glazes on pottery ware

Good to go:
- ∞ stainless steel
- ∞ glass
- ∞ pyrex
- ∞ enamel
- ∞ earthenware
- ∞ cast iron

I'm a big fan of the *Le Creuset* range of cookware. It's an investment, but the high price is justified by the fact that they're awesome to cook with. They are cast iron with a heavy base, so no steam is released and all of your nutrients are retained.

∞ SHOPPING LIST

Veggies

Kale
Silverbeet
Cos lettuce
Spinach
Green capsicum
Red capsicum
Red cabbage
Green cabbage
Zucchini
Onion
Potatoes
Sweet potato
Pumpkin
Corn

Asparagus
Tomatoes
Broccoli
Cucumber
Celery
Brussels sprouts
Cauliflower
Green beans
Leeks
Artichokes
Mushrooms

Fruit

Green apples
Bananas
Kiwi fruit
Lemon
Lime
Sultanas/raisins
Berries
Papaya
Grapes
Figs
Pineapple
Oranges
Mangoes
Watermelon
Cherries
Avocado

Grains
Brown rice
Wild rice
Quinoa
Rolled oats
Oatmeal
Buckwheat
Spelt flour

Legumes
Chickpeas
Brown lentils
Red lentils
Kidney beans

Condiments
Raw apple cider vinegar
Flaxseed oil
Coconut oil
Fresh herbs: basil, dill, coriander, rosemary, sage, thyme,
parsley, oregano
Spices: garlic, turmeric, cayenne, cumin, curry, chilli, ginger,
cinnamon
Almond butter
Tahini
Hummus

Sweeteners
Raw honey
Maple syrup

Stevia
Dates
Coconut sugar
Coconut nectar

Snacks
Popcorn
Raw nuts and seeds

Other
Coconut water

Superfoods
Cacao powder
Cacao nibs
Bee pollen
Maca powder
Spirulina
Chia seeds
Goji berries
Hemp seeds

Aim to buy organic and local produce where possible. If you eat meat, choose organic and grass-finished.

∞ WHERE TO BUY
You should be able to pick up most of the ingredients here from your local supermarket, organic store or farmers' market. You can also look for some of the superfoods online. Here are a few websites I recommend:

Australia
http://lovingearth.net/
http://raw-pleasure.com.au/
http://www.powersuperfoods.com.au/

US
http://www.longevitywarehouse.com/

∞ MAKING FOOD FUN

If you want to make healthy eating sustainable, you have to make it fun. And trust me, it can be so much fun! As I've mentioned, before I became a wellness warrior, I couldn't cook. I've always loved eating, but cooking didn't appeal to me. This is because I hadn't yet become acquainted with the healing magic of food—that eating it can fix what ails you, and that preparing it can be therapeutic. Now, I love to cook. It's a form of meditation for me, as it allows me to get out of my head, follow my intuition, and connect with Mother Nature's gifts. When you think about cooking like that, how can you not love it?

One of the surest ways to make food fun is to not take it too seriously. I think people are so afraid of 'stuffing up' or 'doing something wrong' in the kitchen that it can prevent them from having a go. The thing is, it doesn't matter if something doesn't turn out the way you'd planned it to. Be creative when it comes to flavours, use your intuition when it comes to ingredients, make a mess, and stray from the recipe a little. It's all part of the process of feeling your way in the kitchen and becoming comfortable putting together tasty, healthy dishes. I love experimenting with herbs, spices and ingredients I've never used before, even essential oils. A few drops of peppermint or sweet orange oil in a chocolate recipe is life-changing (just be sure to always use organic and therapeutic food grade oils).

I can't write a book about making peace with your plate without mentioning the most important element in the process—infusing your food with love. This is why eating foods that have been grown by loving hands (either in your own backyard or by a local farmer) is so beneficial. It's also why eating from your own kitchen, and preparing loving meals for yourself and your family, is so important. Be mindful as you're preparing meals. Take time to send gratitude to the ingredients you're working with, for being so damn nutritious. It might sound silly, but this simple step carries so much power.

ᴼᴼᴼᴼᴼ MAKING PEACE WITH LEAVING THE HOUSE

My friends tease me because I carry an esky around with me pretty much whenever I leave the house. If I'm going somewhere and I know I won't be able to get organic food, I make sure I've got a healthy supply with me in my esky. I do this when I'm going to a friend's place, if I'm going shopping, and even if I'm going out for lunch or dinner somewhere that doesn't serve organic food (I do call ahead first, to make sure this is okay with the restaurant or cafe owner). There are two things that make me grumpy: being tired and being hungry. There's nothing worse than going somewhere and not being able to eat anything, so I always make sure the latter doesn't happen by planning ahead and packing an esky.

You may not want to go as far as packing your own food with you wherever you go. If you do need to eat out and you can't get super clean food, simply just do the best you can. If you feel uncomfortable taking your own food to a dinner party or a barbecue, just eat what you're served. In all of these instances, just roll with the moment and don't beat yourself up for it. The guilt that you put on yourself for eating something outside the realm of your new peaceful approach will do more damage than the food anyway.

I want to make a note here about cafes and restaurants that claim to be 'organic'. It's important that we as consumers take responsibility for what we're putting in our bodies by questioning whether the food they're dishing up is really completely organic. I've fallen for this trickery a number of times, and it left me feeling dirty. There's a lot of corruption in the organic world, and a lot of eateries claim to be organic, when in actual fact they serve conventional food with some organic in the mix. It's wrong and deceitful and really pisses me off. So before you get excited about seeing the words "organic" and "café" together, make sure that the café is true to its word. The more we do this, the more the sneaky ones will get the picture that it's not cool to lead us on.

~ TRAVEL LIKE A WELLNESS WARRIOR

Now that I've told you how pedantic I am about preparing my food when I leave the house, you can only imagine how far I go when I have to leave the state or the country! There's nothing worse than eating aeroplane and airport food (actually, hospital food is much worse). I don't even consider it food, and would rather fast and go without than have to

MAKE PEACE WITH YOUR PLATE —

eat it. However, as I said before, I'm not a nice person when I'm hungry. So it's a great idea (mostly for those around me) that I plan ahead and pack a large esky full of enough food to last me until I can get my hands on some organic grub.

Most people don't know this, but you can take food with you on a plane. You just can't take liquids that exceed 100ml and, in some cases, you can't take the food back off the plane. But you can take as much food as you like with you, providing it fits within the carry-on baggage size limit.

This is an example of what I pack for a long-haul flight:

- Two containers of quinoa and salad (one for lunch and one for dinner)
- Apple cider vinegar and flaxseed oil for dressing (I put them in little jars, so they don't exceed 100ml)
- Apples
- Celery sticks
- Almond butter (to spread on the apple slices and celery sticks)
- Brazil nuts
- Homemade trail mix made from goji berries, white mulberries, shredded coconut, cacao nibs and almonds
- Some kind of homemade treats, like cacao balls or oatmeal cookies
- Either chia pudding or muesli soaked in coconut yoghurt (for breakfast)
- Peppermint tea bags and a mug, so I don't have to drink from their plastic cups

∞ Spirulina tablets (to give me my fix of greens)

∞ Chlorella tables (to help detox radiation)

I also make sure I take a stainless steel water bottle with me. The tiny plastic ones that they give you on board just don't cut it!

Recipes

CHAPTER EIGHT

∞ Drinks

Juices

▌GERSON GREEN
- ∞ 1 green apple
- ∞ ¼ green capsicum
- ∞ 2 stalks kale
- ∞ 1 stalk Swiss chard
- ∞ 1 stalk silver beet
- ∞ 2 handfuls cos lettuce
- ∞ Small amount of red cabbage

▌GLOWING GREEN
- ∞ 1 green apple
- ∞ 1 cucumber
- ∞ 1 stalk celery
- ∞ 2 stalks kale

∞ 2 handfuls cos lettuce

∞ A sprig of coriander (cilantro) or mint, optional

CARROT + APPLE

∞ 4 medium carrots

∞ 1 green apple

CARROT + APPLE + BEETROOT

∞ 4 medium carrots

∞ 1 green apple

∞ ½ to 1 small beetroot

Put the ingredients for whichever juice you are making through a juicer. A twin-gear, cold-press juicer is the best; but if you only have a centrifugal type that will do just fine as well. If you want to be creative, add a little ginger or lemon juice to your juices.

GINGER, MINT, LEMON TEA (HOT OR COLD)

∞ ½ lemon

∞ 1 handful of fresh mint

∞ Small amount of ginger (to your own taste)

Add ginger, mint and lemon to a plunger or teacup and pour boiling water on top. Allow to infuse before drinking. If you prefer it cold, add ice or chill before drinking.

EASY GREEN ENERGY DRINK

- ~ 2 cups coconut water
- ~ 1 tsp spirulina

Stir or blend spirulina with coconut water. So easy, and way better for you than a can of Red Bull!

NUT MILK

- ~ 1 cup nuts (choose whichever you like—I prefer almonds, cashews or brazil nuts)
- ~ 4 cups water

1. Soak nuts for at least 8 hours, to deactivate the enzyme inhibitors.
2. Add nuts and water to blender and blend on high for about a minute.
3. Pour blended nuts through a nut milk bag into a large jug or bowl. Use your hands to squeeze out all of the liquid.
4. Store in the fridge. The milk will last for about 4 days.

Smoothies

THE WELLNESS WARRIOR

- ~ 1 large stalk of kale (leaves only)
- ~ 1 large cos lettuce leaf
- ~ 1 small leaf of Swiss chard or silver beet
- ~ 1 small frozen banana (or half a large one)

∞ 1 cup coconut water
∞ ½ lemon, juiced
∞ 1 tsp spirulina
∞ 1 tsp bee pollen
∞ ½ tsp maca powder

1. Wash and prep all ingredients.
2. Chop frozen banana into chunks.
3. Add everything to blender and whiz until smooth.
4. Top up with coconut water or water, if needed.
5. Serve immediately.

GORGEOUS GREENS

∞ 1 large stalk of kale (leaves only)
∞ 1 large cos lettuce leaf
∞ ½ cucumber
∞ 1 stalk celery
∞ 1 small frozen banana (or half a large one)
∞ 1 cup coconut water
∞ 1 sprig of fresh coriander (optional)
∞ 1 tsp spirulina
∞ 1 tsp bee pollen
∞ ½ tsp maca powder

1. Wash and prep all ingredients.
2. Chop frozen banana into chunks.
3. Add everything to blender and whiz until smooth.
4. Top up with coconut water or water, if needed.
5. Serve immediately.

BREAKFAST SUPER SMOOTHIE

- 1 frozen banana
- 1 cup nut milk or coconut milk
- 1 tbs almond butter
- 1 handful of frozen or fresh blueberries
- 1 tsp bee pollen
- 1 tsp maca powder
- 1 tbs chia seeds
- 1 tsp hemp seeds

1. Wash and prep all ingredients.
2. Chop frozen banana into chunks.
3. Add everything to blender and whiz until smooth.
4. Serve immediately.

CHOC-BERRY

- 1 small frozen banana (or half a large one)
- ½ cup frozen mixed berries
- 1 cup coconut water
- 1 tsp bee pollen
- ½ tsp maca powder
- 1 tsp cacao powder
- 1 tsp cacao nibs

1. Chop frozen banana into chunks.
2. Add everything to blender and whiz until smooth.
3. Top up with coconut water or water, if needed.

MINTY FRESH

- 1 handful of cos lettuce
- 1 handful of baby spinach or kale
- ½ frozen banana
- 1 handful of frozen berries
- 1 handful of fresh mint leaves
- 1 tsp chlorella
- 1 tsp bee pollen
- 1 tsp maca
- 1 tsp hemp seeds
- 1 cup coconut water

1. **Chop frozen banana into chunks.**
2. **Add everything to blender and whiz until smooth.**
3. **Top up with coconut water or water, if needed.**

THE KIWI WARRIOR

- 1 large stalk of kale (leaves only)
- 1 large cos lettuce leaf
- 1 small leaf of Swiss chard or silver beet
- ½ frozen banana
- ½ kiwi fruit
- 1 cup coconut water
- ½ lemon, juiced
- 1 tsp spirulina
- 1 tsp bee pollen
- ½ tsp maca powder

1. **Wash and prep all ingredients.**

2. Chop frozen banana into chunks.
3. Add everything to blender and whiz until smooth.
4. Top up with coconut water or water, if needed.
5. Serve immediately.

THE MANGO WARRIOR

- 1 large stalk of kale (leaves only)
- 1 large cos lettuce leaf
- 1 small leaf of Swiss chard or silver beet
- ½ frozen banana
- A few chunks of mango (fresh or frozen)
- 1 cup coconut water
- ½ lemon, juiced
- 1 tsp spirulina
- 1 tsp bee pollen
- ½ tsp maca powder

1. Wash and prep all ingredients.
2. Chop frozen banana into chunks.
3. Add everything to blender and whiz until smooth.
4. Top up with coconut water or water, if needed.
5. Serve immediately.

THE BERRY WARRIOR

- 1 large stalk of kale (leaves only)
- 1 large cos lettuce leaf
- 1 small leaf of Swiss chard or silver beet
- ½ frozen banana

- 1 handful of frozen berries (blueberries, blackberries, raspberries or a mix)
- 1 small handful goji berries
- 1 cup coconut water
- ½ lemon, juiced
- 1 tsp spirulina
- 1 tsp bee pollen
- ½ tsp maca powder

1. Wash and prep all ingredients.
2. Chop frozen banana into chunks.
3. Add everything to blender and whiz until smooth.
4. Top up with coconut water or water, if needed.
5. Serve immediately.

THE PAPAYA WARRIOR

- 1 large stalk of kale (leaves only)
- 1 large cos lettuce leaf
- 1 small leaf of Swiss chard or silver beet
- ½ frozen banana
- A few chunks of papaya (fresh or frozen)
- 1 cup coconut water
- ½ lemon, juiced
- 1 tsp spirulina
- 1 tsp bee pollen
- ½ tsp maca powder

1. Wash and prep all ingredients.
2. Chop frozen banana into chunks.

3. Add everything to blender and whiz until smooth.
4. Top up with coconut water or water, if needed.
5. Serve immediately.

THE LYCHEE WARRIOR

- 1 large stalk of kale (leaves only)
- 1 large cos lettuce leaf
- 1 small leaf of Swiss chard or silver beet
- ½ frozen banana
- 2 lychees (seeds removed)
- 1 cup coconut water
- ½ lemon, juiced
- 1 tsp spirulina
- 1 tsp bee pollen
- ½ tsp maca powder

1. Wash and prep all ingredients.
2. Chop frozen banana into chunks.
3. Add everything to blender and whiz until smooth.
4. Top up with coconut water or water, if needed.
5. Serve immediately.

THE CHOCOLATE WARRIOR

- 1 large stalk of kale (leaves only)
- 1 large cos lettuce leaf
- 1 small leaf of Swiss chard or silver beet
- 1 frozen banana
- 1 cup coconut water

∾ ½ lemon, juiced
∾ 1 tsp cacao
∾ 1 tsp bee pollen
∾ ½ tsp maca powder

1. Wash and prep all ingredients.
2. Chop frozen banana into chunks.
3. Add everything to blender and whiz until smooth.
4. Top up with coconut water or water, if needed.
5. Serve immediately.

NICE TO 'C' YOU (LOADED WITH VITAMIN C)
∾ 1 large stalk of kale (leaves only)
∾ 1 large cos lettuce leaf
∾ 1 small leaf of Swiss chard or silver beet
∾ A few chunks of papaya (fresh or frozen)
∾ ¼ kiwi fruit
∾ 1 small handful of goji berries
∾ 3 lychees
∾ 1 cup coconut water
∾ ½ lemon, juiced
∾ 1 tsp spirulina
∾ 1 tsp bee pollen
∾ ½ tsp maca powder

1. Wash and prep all ingredients.
2. Chop frozen banana into chunks.
3. Add everything to blender and whiz until smooth.

4. Top up with coconut water or water, if needed.
5. Serve immediately.

CHOCOLATE MILKSHAKE
- 2 cups of nut milk
- ½ frozen banana
- 1 handful of frozen blueberries
- 1 heaped tsp cacao powder
- 1 tsp cacao nibs
- Your choice of sweetener to taste (honey, maple syrup, stevia)

Blend all ingredients and serve immediately.

Breakfast

ROLLED OATS
- ¾ cup rolled oats
- 1 cup purified water
- Sultanas (soaked)
- Banana, kiwi fruit, cherries, berries, apple or other fruit of your choice
- Honey
- 1 tsp bee pollen
- 1 tsp chia seeds

1. Put rolled oats in a pot and cover with water.

2. Bring to the boil, simmer for about 10-15 minutes until oats are at desired consistency. You may need to add more water as it is cooking.
3. Top with honey, sultanas, bee pollen, chia seeds and fruit.

QUINOA BREAKFAST PUDDING
- ½ cup quinoa
- 1 green apple
- 1 tbs maple syrup
- 1 tsp almond butter
- 1 tsp cinnamon
- 1 handful of coconut flakes
- 1 handful of almonds

1. Rinse and drain quinoa before cooking in two cups of water. Bring to the boil and simmer for 15-20 minutes, until the water is absorbed.
2. Peel and chop apple into cubes. Add to a saucepan with a little water and cook on medium until slightly soft.
3. Add quinoa, maple syrup, cinnamon, almonds and coconut flakes. Stir to combine and warm through.

APPLE CHIA PUDDING
- 2 tbs chia seeds
- ½ cup coconut water

- 1 green apple
- 2 Medjool dates
- 1 tsp almond butter
- 1 tsp cinnamon
- ½ tsp maca powder (optional)

1. Soak chia seeds in coconut water. Stir, allow to sit for about 15 minutes to form a gel, and then stir occasionally to avoid clumping.
2. Peel and chop apple into cubes. Add to a saucepan with a little water and cook on medium until slightly soft.
3. Add dates and cinnamon to the apples.
4. Stir almond butter and maca powder through the chia seeds.
5. Add apple, dates and cinnamon to the chia gel mixture and combine.
6. Sprinkle a little more cinnamon over the top to serve.

DIY MUESLI

- ½ cup rolled oats
- 1 tbs chia seeds
- 2 tbs coconut flakes
- 1 tbs goji berries
- 1 tbs white mulberries
- 1 tbs bee pollen
- 1 tbs pepitas or sunflower seeds

- ∞ 1 tbs chopped nuts (almond, cashew, brazil, pistachios—or a combo)
- ∞ 1 cup nut milk or coconut milk
- ∞ Cinnamon to sprinkle

1. Combine all dry ingredients in a bowl (you could also have this pre-combined and stored in a glass jar).
2. Pour milk over the muesli.
3. Sprinkle cinnamon on top.

∞ Salads

QUINOA AND TOASTED COCONUT SALAD

- ∞ 1 cup quinoa
- ∞ 1 carrot, diced
- ∞ 1 stalk celery, finely chopped
- ∞ 2 radish, sliced
- ∞ ½ red capsicum, diced
- ∞ ½ green capsicum, diced
- ∞ 1 handful of pistachio nuts
- ∞ 1 handful of walnuts
- ∞ 1 handful of coconut flakes, toasted
- ∞ 1 handful of fresh coriander, roughly chopped
- ∞ Flaxseed oil
- ∞ Lemon juice

1. Rinse and drain quinoa before cooking in two cups of water. Bring to the boil, then simmer for about 15-20 minutes, or until the water is absorbed.
2. Wash and prepare the salad ingredients.
3. Combine all ingredients in a large bowl, and drizzle with lemon juice and flaxseed oil to serve.

BABY SPINACH AND QUINOA SALAD

- 1 cup quinoa
- 1 packet of baby spinach (or enough to feed however many mouths you have)
- 1 red capsicum, thinly sliced
- 1 cup snow peas
- ½ cup walnuts
- ½ cup pistachio nuts
- Flaxseed oil

1. Rinse and drain quinoa before cooking in two cups of water. Bring to the boil, and then simmer for about 15-20 minutes or until the water is absorbed.
2. Wash and prepare the salad ingredients.
3. Combine all ingredients in a large bowl, and drizzle with flaxseed oil to serve.

GARDEN SALAD
- Cos lettuce (enough to feed however many mouths you have)
- 1 carrot
- 1 tomato
- ½ red capsicum
- ½ green capsicum
- ¼ red cabbage
- ½ red onion
- ¼ cup fresh coriander
- Flaxseed oil
- Apple cider vinegar

1. **Wash and prepare all ingredients.**
2. **Combine all ingredients in a large bowl, and drizzle with flaxseed oil and apple cider vinegar to serve.**

QUINOA AND ASPARAGUS SALAD
- 1 packet of mixed lettuce (or enough to feed however many mouths you have)
- 1 cup quinoa
- 1 bunch of asparagus
- ¼ pumpkin, roasted
- 1 zucchini, thinly sliced or spiralled using a spiraliser
- 1 stalk celery, chopped
- 2 radishes, sliced
- ¼ red cabbage
- A few broccoli florets

- ∾ 1 handful of fresh chickpeas
- ∾ ½ cup snow peas
- ∾ 1 small carrot
- ∾ Flaxseed oil
- ∾ Apple cider vinegar

1. Rinse and drain quinoa before cooking in two cups of water. Bring to the boil, and then simmer for about 15-20 minutes, or until the water is absorbed.
2. Chop bottoms off asparagus spears, place in a frying pan and dry fry on low heat for about 15 minutes. Watch and turn every now and then, to prevent burning.
3. Wash and prepare the salad ingredients.
4. Combine all ingredients in a large bowl, and drizzle with flaxseed oil and apple cider vinegar to serve.

ROASTED VEGGIE SALAD
- ∾ A handful of cos lettuce
- ∾ A handful of rocket
- ∾ A handful of kale
- ∾ 1 tomato, sliced
- ∾ 1 red capsicum, sliced
- ∾ 1 carrot, chopped
- ∾ ½ red onion, sliced
- ∾ ¼ red cabbage, chopped
- ∾ ½ eggplant

- ¼ pumpkin
- 1 bunch of asparagus
- Apple cider vinegar
- Flaxseed oil

1. Chop eggplant and pumpkin into chunks, arrange in a baking dish and bake in an oven heated to 180°C for about 45 minutes.
2. Chop bottoms off asparagus spears, place in a frying pan and dry fry on low heat for about 15 minutes. Watch and turn every now and then to prevent burning.
3. Wash and chop all other salad ingredients and combine in a large salad bowl.
4. Plate up the salad, top with roast veggies and asparagus. Serve with apple cider vinegar and flaxseed oil.

Hearty meals

SPICED BAKED POTATOES

- 4 potatoes
- 1 tbs coconut oil
- 1 tsp turmeric
- 1 tsp cumin
- 1 tsp cayenne pepper

1. Wash/scrub potatoes and chop into cubes.

2. Arrange on a baking dish and coat with coconut oil.
3. Sprinkle spices over the top and roll potato cubes in them to coat.
4. Bake in an oven heated to 180°C for about an hour.

BOK CHOY ROLLS
- 1 cup brown rice
- ⅛ cup wild rice
- 1 cob of corn (slice kernels off cob)
- ½ capsicum, finely chopped
- ½ brown onion, finely chopped
- 1 cup peas
- 12 extra large bok choy leaves
- ¾ cup honey
- ½ cup lemon juice

1. Soak rice for 8 hours. Rinse and strain.
2. Cook rice using the absorption method. One part rice, two parts water, bring to the boil and then reduce to simmer, until all of the water has been absorbed and the rice is cooked. Once cooked, strain and run hot water through it.
3. In a bowl, combine rice, corn, peas, capsicum and brown onion.
4. Spoon mixture into the centre of a bok choy leaf and wrap like a parcel. Repeat for all 12 leaves.

5. Place parcels in a baking dish with the smooth side up and the folded sides tucked underneath. Fill the dish to make the parcels snug.
6. Drizzle a generous amount of honey and lemon juice over the parcels and the bottom of the dish.
7. Bake for 30 minutes in a low to moderate oven (160°C to 180° C).
8. Serve using a spatula.

BROWN RICE VEGGIE PATTIES
(makes 11 patties)

- 1 cup brown rice
- ½ large sweet potato
- ¼ pumpkin
- 3 potatoes
- 1 tsp curry powder
- 1 tsp cumin
- 1 tsp turmeric
- 1 clove garlic
- 1 tbs fresh coriander
- Rye flour (or whatever type of flour you prefer)

1. Soak rice for 8 hours to deactivate the enzyme inhibitors.
2. Peel potatoes, pumpkin and sweet potato and cut into chunks.
3. Roast veggies in an oven heated to 180°C for about an hour.

4. Add rice to a pot with two cups of water. Bring to the boil, and then reduce to simmer for 40 minutes, or until the water has been absorbed and the rice is cooked.
5. Once veggies are cooked, either mash by hand or use a blender or food processor to combine them. Add garlic, coriander and spices to the mix.
6. Combine rice and veggie mix together in a large bowl; add a little flour to bind the mixture.
7. Use your hands to form the patties and arrange on a baking dish (or two).
8. Bake patties in an oven heated to 180°C for about 40 mins, or until browned.
9. Serve with salad and satay sauce (recipe below).

FOR THE SATAY SAUCE:

- 2 tbs almond butter
- Juice of 1 lime
- 2 tsp hemp seeds
- 2 tbs flaxseed oil
- 2 tsp apple cider vinegar
- 1 clove garlic

Blend all ingredients together.

LENTIL COCONUT CURRY

- 3 cups shredded coconut
- 1½ cups French lentils

- ∞ 3-4 tsp organic curry powder (I look for one without salt)
- ∞ 1 onion
- ∞ 3 cloves garlic
- ∞ 2 small carrots (or one large)
- ∞ 1 zucchini
- ∞ 1 cup broccoli
- ∞ 1 capsicum (aka bell pepper)
- ∞ 1 sweet potato
- ∞ 1 large potato
- ∞ 1 large tomato
- ∞ Coriander (aka cilantro) to taste

FOR THE COCONUT MILK:

(I make my own coconut milk because it is super easy to do, and all of the canned ones seem to contain guar gum. If you're up for it, I totally suggest making your own.)

1. Blend 3 cups of shredded coconut with 6 cups of water over high heat for a couple of minutes.
2. Use a nut milk bag, cheesecloth, or a tea towel draped over a mesh strainer to strain the milk.
3. Squeeze the bag to make sure you extract all of the milk.

FOR THE CURRY:

1. Heat garlic and onion in a pot (with coconut oil if you like). Add curry powder and mix for a couple of seconds.

2. Add lentils to the pot and combine with onion and spices.
3. Add coconut milk to the pot and bring to the boil. Once boiling, reduce to simmer for about 20 minutes.
4. Add the rest of the vegetables and continue to simmer for another 20 minutes, or until veggies and lentils are cooked. Lentils should be soft, but still retain their shape.
5. Serve topped with fresh coriander.

SIMPLE QUINOA + VEG
- 1 cup quinoa
- 1 zucchini
- 1 carrot
- 1-2 handfuls of snow peas
- 1 cup broccoli
- 1-2 handfuls of baby spinach
- 2 cloves garlic
- 1 lemon, juiced

1. Rinse and drain your quinoa.
2. Add quinoa to a pot with two cups of water. Bring to the boil, and then reduce to simmer for about 15 minutes, or until all of the water has been absorbed.
3. While that's cooking, chop up all of your veggies.

4. Once quinoa is cooked, add all veggies (except baby spinach) to the pot, along with garlic and lemon juice.
5. Stir veggies through, and cook on low until they are as cooked as you like them. I prefer my veggies crunchy, so I just barely give them time to warm through.
6. At the last minute, throw in the baby spinach and give it all a stir through.
7. Serve!

SATAY NOODLES
(makes 2 serves)
- 2 large zucchinis
- 1 large tomato
- 1 carrot
- 2 radishes
- 1 red capsicum
- 1 small onion
- 1 handful of coconut flakes
- 1 handful of pistachio nuts

FOR THE SATAY SAUCE:
- 2 tbs almond butter
- Juice of 1 lime
- 2 tsp hemp seeds
- 2 tsb flaxseed oil
- 2 tsp apple cider vinegar
- 1 clove garlic

1. Turn the zucchinis into noodles using a *Spirooli* or spiralising tool.
2. Prepare and slice the rest of the veggies and combine with noodles.
3. Combine ingredients for the sauce in a blender.
4. Pour sauce over the noodles and serve.

VEGGIE SHEPHERD'S PIE

- 1 cup brown lentils
- 1 brown onion
- 1 red capsicum
- 1 stalk celery
- 4 cloves garlic, crushed
- 2 tsp ginger, grated
- 1 small chilli
- 2 tsp cumin
- 1 tsp coriander powder
- 1 zucchini
- 2 potatoes
- 4 large tomatoes
- 2 cups of veggie stock
- Coconut oil

1. Boil potatoes, then mash and set aside for later.
2. Heat coconut oil in a pot and add garlic, ginger, onion, cumin and coriander.
3. Add lentils and stir through spices.

4. Add veggie stock and bring to the boil. Once boiling, reduce to medium heat.

5. Add celery and capsicum, then reduce to simmer for about 30 minutes, or until most of the liquid has been absorbed.

6. Add tomatoes and stir through. Allow to simmer for another 10-15 minutes, until most of the liquid has been absorbed.

7. Transfer lentils to a baking dish. Top with slices of zucchini and mashed potato.

8. Bake in an oven heated to 180°C, until the potato starts to brown on top.

PIZZA

FOR THE BASE:

- 2 cups flour (rye, buckwheat or spelt)
- 2 tsp baking powder
- 2 tbp chia seeds
- ¼ cup coconut oil
- ¾ cup water

FOR THE TOPPING:

- 4 cloves garlic
- 3 tomatoes
- 1 zucchini
- ⅛ pumpkin
- 1 capsicum
- 1 avocado

- 1 brown onion
- Nutritional yeast
- Herbs of your choice (I use basil, oregano, rosemary, thyme)

1. Preheat the oven to 180°C.
2. Make the base by combing all ingredients, and kneading until they form a dough-like consistency. Cover your bench with extra flour, then use a rolling pin to roll out the pizza base.
3. Grease a pan with coconut oil, and then press the dough into your pizza shape.
4. Bake dough for about 15-20 minutes (depending on how thick it is).
5. Take the half-cooked dough out of the oven, then dress it with your pizza toppings. Spread avocado, garlic and some herbs on the base, then layer on thin slices of tomatoes and vegetables.
6. Bake dressed pizza for another 15 minutes, until the toppings are cooked and the crust is browned.
7. Sprinkle extra herbs and nutritional yeast on top.
8. Slice and serve!

VEGGIE BAKE
- 2 potatoes
- ½ sweet potato
- 1 ½ zucchini
- 6 tomatoes
- ⅛ pumpkin

- 1 eggplant
- 1 cup mushrooms
- 1 onion
- 4 garlic cloves, crushed
- A handful of fresh basil, roughly chopped
- ½ cup cashews (soaked for a few hours)
- 2-3 tbs nutritional yeast
- Juice of half a lemon
- 1 tsp apple cider vinegar

1. Pre-heat oven to 180°C.
2. Thinly slice veggies and layer them in a large baking dish. I like to layer in this order: potato, sweet potato, eggplant, ½ of the tomato, ½ of the garlic, ½ of the basil, mushrooms, pumpkin, zucchini. Pop in the oven and cook for about 40 minutes.
3. Take out of the oven and add the other ½ of the tomaoto, Bake for another 10 minutes.
4. Combine these ingredients for the "cheese" sauce in a blender, adding water if necessary to obtain a creamy consistency: cashews, lemon juice, apple cider vinegar, 2 garlic cloves, basil.
5. Pour sauce over the top of the veggies, and bake for another 5-10 minutes.

∞∞∞ Sweets

⁞ CASHEW CREAM
- ∞∞∞ 1 cup cashews
- ∞∞∞ 1 tsp maple syrup

1. Soak cashews in water for eight hours.
2. Strain cashews and blend with maple syrup until smooth.

⁞ RAW CHOCOLATE
- ∞∞∞ 110g raw almonds or brazil nuts
- ∞∞∞ 1 cup coconut oil
- ∞∞∞ 4 tbs cacao powder
- ∞∞∞ 1 handful of medjool dates, chopped
- ∞∞∞ ¼ cup of coconut nectar
- ∞∞∞ 1 handful of shredded coconut
- ∞∞∞ 1 handful of goji berries
- ∞∞∞ 1 handful of frozen raspberries

1. Line a medium-sized baking dish with non-stick paper. Place in the freezer to chill while you mix up the ingredients.
2. Grind almonds in a blender or food processor until they are fairly fine (not a powder though).
3. Blend coconut oil, cacao and coconut syrup.
4. Stir through chopped nut, goji berries, shredded coconut and raspberries.

5. Pour the mixture into the dish, making sure it spreads out thinly and evenly.
6. Put into the freezer until it has set, and then keep in the freezer between pig outs.

▌ CHOC-CHIA PUDDING
(1 serving)

- ∞ 2 tbs chia seeds
- ∞ ½ cup coconut water (or nut milk)
- ∞ 1 tbs cacao powder
- ∞ 1 tsp cacao nibs
- ∞ 1 tsp raw honey (or maple syrup)
- ∞ 1 tsp shredded coconut
- ∞ 1 tsp almond butter
- ∞ 1 handful of blueberries

1. Combine chia seeds and coconut water and stir well. Let it sit for about 10 minutes while the seeds soak up the water, stirring a few times to avoid clumping.
2. Stir in the rest of the ingredients.
3. Allow the mixture to sit and thicken to your desired consistency.

▌ RAW CHOC-GOJI BROWNIES

- ∞ 1 cup whole walnuts
- ∞ 1¼ cups Medjool dates, pitted
- ∞ ½ cup raw cacao

- ½ cup raw unsalted almonds, roughly chopped
- ¼ cup goji berries

1. Place walnuts in food processor and blend on high, until the nuts are finely ground.
2. Add the cacao and pulse to combine.
3. Add the dates one at a time through the feed tube of the food processor while it is running. What you should end up with is a mix that appears rather like cake crumbs but, when pressed, will easily stick together. (If the mixture does not hold together well, add more dates.)
4. In a large bowl, combine the walnut-cacao mix with the chopped almonds and goji berries.
5. Press into cake pan or dish. Place in freezer or fridge until ready to serve. (It is also easier to cut these when they are very cold.) Store in an airtight container.

APPLE PUDDING

FOR THE BASE:

- 200g walnuts
- 75g desiccated coconut
- 80g Medjool dates
- 1 tbs coconut oil
- 1 tbs honey
- 1 tbs cinnamon

1. Blend the walnuts until there are no big chunks. Add the rest of the ingredients and blend to a dough-like consistency.
2. Spoon mixture into a baking dish and spread evenly over the base.

FOR THE APPLE FILLING:

- ∞∞ 3 large green apples
- ∞∞ 2 bananas
- ∞∞ 100g chia seeds
- ∞∞ 1 tbs honey
- ∞∞ 1 tbs coconut oil
- ∞∞ 1 tbs cinnamon
- ∞∞ Juice of ½ lemon

1. Blend one of the apples with the bananas, chia seeds, lemon juice and honey. Set aside for 15 minutes to form a gel.
2. Slice the remaining two apples. Cover the crust with half the apples and sprinkle with cinnamon.
3. Spoon the chia gel mixture on top of the apple slices, then place the rest of the sliced apples on top. Sprinkle the top with cinnamon and a drizzle of coconut oil.
4. Bake in an oven heated to 150°C for 25-30 minutes.

RICE PUDDING
- 1 cup brown rice
- 2 cups almond milk
- ½ cup Medjool dates, chopped and seeds removed
- 2 tbs sultanas
- ¼ cup maple syrup
- 2 tsp cinnamon

1. Soak rice for 8 hours, to deactivate the enzyme inhibitors.
2. Add rice and almond milk to a pot. Bring to the boil, and then reduce to simmer for about 45 minutes or until the rice is cooked.
3. When rice is cooked, add dates, cinnamon and maple syrup and stir through.
4. Serve warm with a sprinkling of extra cinnamon.

LEMON AND COCONUT CAKE
- 2 cups rye flour (or flour of your choice)
- 1 cup desiccated coconut
- 1 tsp yeast
- Juice of two lemons
- Rind of one lemon
- 1 banana, mashed
- ¼ pear, grated
- 2 tbs chia seeds
- ½ cup coconut water (or water)
- 2 tbs coconut oil
- 4 Medjool dates, de-seeded and chopped
- ¼ cup maple syrup

ICING INGREDIENTS:

- 1 cup cashews
- 2 tsp desiccated coconut
- Juice of two lemons
- 1 tbs maple syrup

For the cake:

1. Mix chia seeds with the coconut water (or water) to form a gel (this acts as an egg replacer).
2. Combine all ingredients in a large mixing bowl.
3. Spoon mixture into a baking dish.
4. Bake in an oven (preheated to 180°C) for an hour.
5. Once cooked, remove from the oven and allow to cool down before icing.

For the icing:

1. Soak the cashews for at least an hour.
2. Combine cashews, coconut, lemon juice and maple syrup in a blender; whiz until smooth.
3. Spread icing over the cake.

CHEESECAKE

- 2 cups of raw cashews (soaked, rinsed, drained)
- 1 cup of almond meal
- ¾ cup of dates (de-pitted)
- Juice of 1½ lemons

- ∞ ¼ cup maple syrup
- ∞ Mixed berries to serve

For the crust:

1. Blend almond meal and dates together.
2. Press mixture into baking dish.

For the 'cheese' filling:

1. Blend cashews, lemon juice and maple syrup until smooth.
2. Spoon the filling on top of the crust.
3. Freeze for at least an hour before serving.
4. Serve with mixed berries.

AVOCADO COCONUT LIME CHEESECAKE

FOR THE CRUST:

- ∞ Blend 1 cup of almond meal with ¾ cup of Medjool dates; then press into a pie dish.

FOR THE FILLING:

- ∞ 2 medium/large avocados
- ∞ 6 tbs honey
- ∞ ½ cup lime juice
- ∞ 5 tbs melted coconut oil
- ∞ ½ cup shredded coconut

1. Blend all ingredients and spoon on top of the crust.
2. Transfer dish to fridge or freezer, until it has set firm.

CHOCOLATE CHEESECAKE

FOR THE CRUST:

Blend 1 cup of almond meal with ¾ cup of Medjool dates; then press into a pie dish.

FOR THE FILLING:

- 1 cup cashews
- 1 frozen banana
- ½ avocado
- ¼ cup maple syrup (or more if you want it sweeter)
- 2 tbs cacao powder

1. Blend all ingredients and spoon on top of the crust.
2. Transfer dish to fridge or freezer, until it has set firm.

OAT COOKIES WITH JAM AND CREAM

FOR THE COOKIES:

- 1 cup rolled oats
- 1 cup oatmeal
- 2 carrots (grated)

- ½ cup shredded coconut
- A little coconut oil (just enough to add moisture)
- 1 tbs chia seeds (made into a gel with about ¼ cup water)

Combine ingredients, form into balls, and then bake in an oven heated to 180°C for between 45 mins and 1 hour.

FOR THE JAM:

(This is an estimate. My Dad and I made this jam one Sunday afternoon and didn't measure anything, so use your instincts with this one.)

- 3 cups strawberries
- 1 cup honey
- 1 grated apple
- 1 tbs lemon juice

Add ingredients to a large pot over high heat. Once the mixture boils, lower the heat to medium and boil lightly for 30 to 60 minutes. Scrape the sides of the pot and stir as you go. The longer the jam cooks, the thicker the final product will be.

For the cream:

Blend 1 cup cashews (soaked for a few hours) with 1 tsp maple syrup (or more if you like it sweet).

LEMON COCONUT SLICE

FOR THE BASE:

- ¾ cup rolled oats
- ¾ cup dates
- ¾ cup shredded coconut

Blend oats and coconut. Add the dates and process until it all sticks together. Press into the bottom of a square baking dish and then put in the fridge.

FOR THE FILLING:

- ⅓ cup melted coconut oil
- ¼ cup maple syrup or coconut nectar
- Juice of 3 lemons
- 2 bananas
- ½ cup shredded coconut

Blend all the ingredients until smooth, and then pour the mixture over the base layer. Leave the slice in the fridge overnight to set (or even in the freezer for a while, if you want it sooner). Cut into slices.

FASTING AND CLEANSING

∞ Digestion takes up so much of our body's energy. As soon as we eat something, energy is diverted away from other areas of our body and rushes to our digestive system, to get to work breaking down and digesting what we've just eaten. The amount of energy that is needed depends on how difficult or easy the item of food is to digest. For instance, fruits and veggies are easy to digest, whole grains and nuts are a little harder, and meat is super hard (meat takes about three days to be properly broken down and pass through).

When we are constantly feeding ourselves, our bodies are constantly in digestion mode and aren't able to do other jobs like healing, repairing and rejuvenating. This is one of the reasons why we do so much healing in our sleep: we aren't eating. It's also why it's a good idea to eat lighter in the evening.

∞ Fun fact

Did you know that, if you had a big meal and then exercised straight after, the food you just ate would not be properly digested? This is because the energy would be diverted to your arms and legs and away from your digestive system. The food would remain in your system waiting to be broken down, and getting all funky in the meantime.

∞ THE 48-HOUR LIQUID FAST

The point of my message is that, when our bodies aren't busy digesting, they can get to work on other important tasks like healing. So, this is why it's a good idea to give your system a break every now and then and solely consume liquids. I'm not saying you have to live on juices (unless you want to), although this is a gentler form of fasting than you may have heard elsewhere. Liquid fasting is like a mini-break for your digestion, and is perfect to do on weekends every now and then.

This is what a 48-hour liquid fast may look like:

∞ First thing in the morning, drink a glass of water followed by a cup of water with lemon juice. It's important to add lemon juice to warm water, not boiling, as boiling water will kill the vitamin C.

∞ Drink at least six glasses of fresh veggie juice each day. You can mix it up, but I prefer to keep the majority of them green.

∞ Drink two green smoothies each day. These can be your meals, for lunch and dinner.

~ If smoothies aren't enough for meals, you could also have a bowl of vegetable soup.

~ Drink other liquids like coconut water (with a teaspoon of spirulina for extra boost), herbal teas and plain purified water.

~ Eat a bowl of chia pudding each day for dessert (hey, who said fasting had to be void of dessert?)

Important bits to know:

~ Just because you're not eating solid food, you shouldn't skimp on nutrients. Make sure that you cram a whole heap of veggies and superfoods into your 48 hours, so that your body is still flooded with goodness.

~ Allow yourself more resting and sleeping while on the fast, to make sure you're giving your body what it needs to make the most of the healing period.

~ When you finish a cleanse or fast, it is important to ease out of it slowly. If you resume eating meat or foods that you know are tough on the digestive system, I recommend gradually working them back in.

~ If your body is pretty toxic, you may experience detox symptoms in the form of headaches, lethargy and nausea. You can give the process a little nudge by eliminating toxins with things like dry body brushing and coffee enemas.

~ You will wee a lot. It's a great idea to stock up on toilet paper.

∞ THE 10-DAY CLEANSE

Now that you're armed with all of this Wellness Warrior knowledge, it's time to put it into practice. What better way to do that than to treat your body to a good ol' internal scrubbing? If you can't make ten days, just do as many as you can. Know that every day your willpower holds, the cleaner and healthier you will be. This cleanse will strip away accumulated crap and provide a blank canvas for you to begin your new healthy lifestyle.

For ten days, you will commit to consuming:

∞ mostly fresh juice
∞ a few smoothies
∞ some salads
∞ as much water and as many herbal teas as you like

∞ WHY CLEANSE?

'Detox' is a bit of a dirty word. This isn't because detoxifying our bodies is a bad idea—very much the opposite, actually. It's because most detoxes are approached in completely the wrong way. They are seen as temporary stages of deprivation, where real food is replaced by powdered crap. And they are usually followed by a reversal back to nasty habits, that will undo any good work.

The purpose of this cleanse is to detoxify your body and dislodge and eliminate sludge and gunk that has been allowed to build up in your system. But it's more than that. It's designed to be a kick-start into a healthy lifestyle. There's not much point in cleansing, if you're just going to put the crap straight back in. Beginning a healthy lifestyle change with a period of intense cleansing will get right into the nitty gritty of your cells. It will shift toxins and allow your body to absorb nutrients more efficiently.

A clean body is a vessel that will boast glowing skin, strong hair, bright eyes and boatloads of energy. You will think more clearly, feel better, and effortlessly find your ideal weight. You will emanate love and vitality from the inside out!

Dealing with detox symptoms

By about the third or fourth day you'll most probably start to feel pretty crappy. This isn't because the cleanse is detrimental to your health (if it's done properly). Seedy symptoms are simply a normal part of the detoxifying process. As toxins are stirred up and released, you may experience headaches, mood swings, crazy emotions, nausea and fatigue. Old injuries may also flare up. If the symptoms become too much to handle, coffee enemas will provide relief.

Preparation

It's a good idea to do some internal homework before you go launching into a full on cleanse. In the week leading up to the cleanse, reduce or eliminate toxins like coffee, cigarettes, alcohol and processed foods. It's also smart to start reducing your dairy, meat, salt and sugar consumption.

Weaning

Once you've made it through the duration of the cleanse, it's important that you don't go out and scoff the first smorgasbord of solid food you can find. The winding down phase is just as important as the preparation phase. Start by introducing salads and some lightly-cooked vegetables. Then introduce whole grains, legumes and beans. If you choose to eat meat, make it a slow reappearance into your diet. Once you've reset your insides with a cleanse, you've got yourself a clean slate to continue with the awesome healthy lifestyle you've learnt about in this book.

THE DAILY ROUTINE

On waking: Drink one tsp of raw apple cider vinegar with the juice of ½ a lemon in warm water

Breakfast: Green smoothie or green juice

Morning snack #1: Juice

Morning snack #2: Juice

Lunch: Juice **or** smoothie, with the option of having a plate of salad with flaxseed oil and apple cider vinegar dressing

Afternoon snack #1: Juice

Afternoon snack #2: Juice or smoothie

Dinner: Juice or smoothie

After dinner: Peppermint tea

Note #1: These are just the minimum juicing requirements. If you would like to drink more, go right ahead!

Note #2: Feel free to drink as much purified water and herbal tea as you like throughout the day.

Note #3: *I have given the option of having a smoothie or a salad where indicated, just in case you feel like an all-juice cleanse is too intense for you. All juice is best, because that way your body is given a break from digesting fibre. But you will get heaps of benefits if you include a smoothie or a little bit of salad, if needed.*

ALL IN YOUR HEAD

PART THREE

GOING BEYOND OUR PLATES

CHAPTER TEN

I believe there is no separation of mind, body and emotions. Thoughts, attitudes and belief systems have an enormous impact on your physical wellbeing. Conversely, if your body is ailing, your mental health will be compromised. All of our body parts are connected and influence each other.

∞∞∞ Dr Frank Lipman

Health and wellness have so much more to them than just food. Have you ever noticed how we tend to turn to food when we're sad, angry, stressed or experiencing any other emotion we don't really want to deal with? It's our method of coping, our way of numbing us out of our reality, and our way of distracting us from our true feelings. Because feelings and raw emotions are bat shit scary, right?

Hell no, they're not! We're just conditioned to think that way. When you consider that all of this emotional eating could be the reason you don't look the way you want in teeny denim shorts, allowing your feelings to sit on the surface doesn't seem so bad. This is easy enough to say; putting it into practice is the tricky part—especially when we've been reliant on food to boost our moods for so long.

This chapter is going to cover some tools for getting the rest of your life in order, so that you don't need chips and ice cream to give you temporary fulfilment, together with lasting cottage cheese thighs.

‱ MEDITATION

Even though meditation is daunting (and snooze inducing) for some people, it's also one of the most effective ways to cultivate a happy life. The main benefit of meditation (apart from delivering calm and serenity) is that it teaches us how to be okay with just being.

When you close your eyes and sit in meditation, with nothing to achieve and nothing to do apart from concentrate on your breathing and the sensations in your body, you quickly learn how to be content without any of the bells and whistles of our busy modern lives. You may hate it at first; you may struggle with the silence and stillness. But trust me when I say that, after a while, you'll notice subtle changes in your everyday life. Your patience and coping mechanisms will improve, you will be easier to please, you will be able to see the bigger picture, and you'll be more content in the present moment. You won't **need** anything else to make you happy—you will be happy for absolutely no other reason than because you are alive in the moment.

Thanks to the endless amount of options we have available to us at any given moment, we're conditioned to fear stillness.

Doing absolutely nothing at all makes us uncomfortable. We move quickly from task to task and, whenever the threat of stillness begins to creep in, we generally dart towards the nearest distraction. It might be checking emails, jumping on social media (scrolling through *Instagram* is my distraction of choice), drinking alcohol, having a cigarette or heading to the fridge. Food is a massive emotional salve but, just like all of these other external solutions, it's temporary and unfulfilling.

No-one likes to feel sad, angry, anxious or any other so-branded 'negative emotion', but it's imperative that we do. When an emotion comes bubbling up to the surface, smothering it with a temporary distraction will only cause it to fester into something much more dramatic, like a disease. Plus, if we discriminate and only allow ourselves to feel positive emotions, we deny ourselves so much magic. It's only by sitting with and feeling our uncomfortable emotions— without labelling them—that we can transcend them and reach the pot of gold (aka priceless wisdom and lessons) on the other side of them. Emotions won't kill us—feeling is healing! And if you really feel into the emotion, whatever is going on inside will only last for 12 minutes before it passes. So, there's really no need to be so afraid of them.

I've been meditating daily for almost four years and I still have a love-hate relationship with it. There are some days when I'm able to sit on my meditation stool and allow my body to blissfully melt into relaxation to the symphony of my breath. Then there are the mornings when all I can focus on is how sore my shoulders are, or whatever work I have to do during the day. When my mind is busy like that, it's a sign that I need to dedicate more time to getting out of it. It's the times that I least feel like meditating when I know it is most beneficial for me.

How to meditate

∞ Schedule a time

I like to meditate first thing in the morning, after I've showered to wake myself up and/or exercised to get myself out of my head and into my body. But others might prefer to do it later in the day or before bed. Do whatever works for you. I've found that meditating at the same time each day helps to create a habit. Habit leads to transformation.

∞ Create a sacred space

I have a special meditation room. In it I have my meditation stool, cushions, blankets, as well as an altar adorned with a candle, crystals and angel cards. Don't worry if you don't have a whole room to spare. You can meditate sitting up in bed, or just in a quiet corner of the house. Again, it helps to create a habit out of meditation, when you have a designated mediation space.

∞ Don't wait until everything is perfect

Who cares if your room isn't set up, you don't have the right stool or cushion, or your house isn't dead quiet? Meditate anyway! Just start wherever you are, with whatever you have. Being able to still the mind amidst chaos is part of the challenge anyway!

∞ Meditate like this …

1. Sit on your meditation stool, cushion or up in bed. Adjust your position so that you are symmetrical, upright, open and a little uncomfortable (if you're

too comfy you could fall asleep). Roll your neck and your shoulders and settle in. I like to wrap a blanket around my waist, so that I have something to rest my hands on in my lap. I find this takes the pressure off my shoulders.

2. Close your eyes and gently focus your attention on the space in front of them, between your eyebrows. This is called your 'Third Eye'—it's said to house all of your intuitive powers.

3. Concentrate on and listen to your breathing. Notice the rise and fall of the abdomen on each inhalation and exhalation. Feel the subtle sensation in the space between your nose and upper lip, as you breathe in and out.

4. Open your awareness to include the sounds around you—outside and inside the room. Listen for birds, cars, people making noises, etc. Just be aware of them, without focusing on them.

5. You'll find your mind will tend to wander. That's okay—it does for even the most seasoned meditator. When it does, just bring your attention back to your breathing and the sounds you hear.

6. Try to sit and keep your mind calm for as long as you can. Start with 5-10 minutes a day, then go up to 15-20 minutes a day, and then go up to 30 minutes or however long you like. The more you practise, the longer you'll be able to hold mental focus.

This above method is called 'mindfulness meditation'. It's one of the best ways to cultivate a peaceful internal environment.

Because there's nothing to do, and nothing to achieve, it forces you to practise living in the present moment. And when you're in the present moment, there's no space for worry, fear or anxiety.

It may seem tricky to begin with. That's because you're not trying to achieve anything besides the ability to be comfortable and content with your own presence. Stick with it and eventually your practice will go from something that seems like a chore, to something you can't go a day without.

Awesome meditation script

Guided meditations can be a great way to ease into a meditation practice. They can help you to escape your thoughts more easily. Record yourself reading out the dialogue below, and use it as a meditation soundtrack:

Sit or lie comfortably. Allow your hands to rest in your lap or beside you, palms upwards. Gently close your eyes. Just take a moment to focus on your breathing, and notice the gentle in and out of your breath.

As you breathe in say to yourself, 'I am' and, as your breath flows out, say 'relaxed' Repeat. Now feel a wave of relaxation flowing from your toes up to your head and then continuing to flow gently through your body.

Allow your mind and thoughts to quieten. If thoughts do come, just let them pass through without any attention to them. Focus back on your breathing: 'I am relaxed'.

If you find that your mind is going back to the same thoughts and stories, gently breathe out and say, 'I let go'.

Divert your attention to the sounds of the birds and trees, and always come back to your breath.

Bring your attention to your feet. Notice the way they feel, feel any sensations that are in them. Now breathe into your feet and, as you exhale, release all tension.

Move your awareness up to your lower legs. Breathe in and contract the muscles in your calves; as you breathe out, release the muscles and completely relax.

Focus your attention on your thighs. Tighten the large muscles as you take a breath in; hold it for a second, before breathing out and relaxing.

Next become aware of how you are feeling in your hips. Are you holding on to any tension or emotion in this area? Take a moment to breathe into your hips; then breathe out, and let go of anything you may be holding on to.

Allow your awareness to move up to your chest. Take a deep breath in, then puff your chest out. Hold it for a moment, before breathing out and completely relaxing. Say to yourself, 'I am relaxed'.

Bring your attention to your throat. How is the energy in this area? Is there anything you are afraid of saying or holding back? If so, breathe into whatever this may be. When you breathe out, release any fear or attachment you may have.

To relax the muscles in your neck and shoulders, bring your shoulders up to your ears, then drop them back down and relax into the chair.

Move your attention up to your face. Tighten all of the muscles in your face. Really scrunch it up. And then gently breathe out, releasing all of the tension and feel your face smooth out and relax.

Focus on the dark space between your eyes. Return to your breathing; gently in and out through the nose. Notice the rise and fall of your chest with each breath in and out.

Recall whether there was anywhere in your body that felt tense or uncomfortable. If you can easily reach it, place your hand on that area. Consciously breathe into that area and, as you do, ask yourself quietly 'Why do I feel this way—what is causing this tension, pain or discomfort in this part of my body?' Then just quieten the mind and allow the answer to come to you.

Visualise a radiant white light around your heart; see it expanding and almost vibrating with love. Now allow this love to flow down your arm and through your hand, into that part of the body where you have any discomfort. Allow this flow of love to continue warming and easing that part of you, then see it flowing throughout your body, visiting and embracing every cell, every muscle and organ with healing love. Gently say to yourself, 'I love and accept myself exactly as I am. I listen to my body's messages with love. I take loving care of my body and my body responds to me with vibrant health and energy. My healing is in process, and all is well in my world'.

Now when you are ready, bring your attention back to the room; take a couple of long, deep breaths and gently crack open your eyes, slowly and mindfully taking in your surroundings.

EXPERT WORD ⦚ DR IAN GAWLER

Meditation reconnects us with our true selves. All of the things we aspire to are actually our natural states. As life goes on, these natural states have layers added to them. As adults, if we haven't learnt how to deal with the difficulties of life, they can overwhelm us and cause us to make poor choices. Meditation re-establishes a natural balance; it teaches us how to relax physically and how to actually get our mind back into this calm and clear state. There's an inner peace that comes with that and leads to a natural self-esteem. That comes out of a sense of connecting with our fundamental goodness. Out of that comes a respect. A lot of people who meditate find that, as the months go by, they naturally gravitate towards eating better because, when you meditate, you become more aware. If you feel good about yourself and you have that inner respect, why would you want to knock it around? It doesn't mean that you can't have fun, but you do it in a way that's actually good for you. Meditation naturally brings out the best in human qualities.

Ian Gawler is one of Australia's most famous long-term cancer survivors and an experienced, respected authority on 'mind-body medicine' and meditation.

⸺ SUNLIGHT

Have you ever wondered why your mood lifts when the sun comes out? Or why it feels so good to lie outside and let your skin soak up some sunshine? It's because the sun is so good for us! We are like plants—the human body needs sunlight to grow, thrive and survive. Sunlight is a vital element of any wellness regime, and it's crucial for preventing illness and maintaining good health.

Despite common sense, there's a lot of confusion around the topic of sunshine. For the past 30 years or so, the sun has been the subject of much demonising. Doctors, dermatologists, health officials, beauty experts, product companies and that darn convincing *Slip, Slop, Slap* bird have had us running for cover the second we feel the heat of the sun on our skin. We are well-educated about the link between skin cancer and sunlight exposure. But, as a result of this over-simplification of facts, we've gone from one extreme to the other.

We're now so afraid of burning that our bodies are becoming severely deprived of vitamin D—a hormone best sourced from the sun. Our bodies use sunlight to help our skin produce the vitamin D it needs to build bones, suppress inflammation, strengthen the immune system and protect against cancer (including skin cancer).

A research paper by internationally-recognised research scientist and vitamin D expert, Dr William Grant PhD, shows just how strong the evidence that sunlight fights cancer really is. His conclusions state that:

> *From a scientific point of view, vitamin D reduces the risk of developing many types of cancer and increases survival, once cancer reaches the detectable stage.*

Six tips for avoiding vitamin D deficiency

1. Get your daily dose of sun
   The best way to increase your vitamin D levels is through safe, smart, limited sunscreen-free exposure to

the sun. Just 20 minutes of sun exposure daily should
be all you need (although this varies depending on
where you live, what type of skin you have and your
age). Never lie out in the sun for extended periods
of time or during the hottest part of the day. Always
avoid sunburn and build up a tolerance to the sun
slowly. If you're fair-skinned, start introducing your
skin to the sun in the cooler months, in the morning
or afternoon.

2. Embrace uninterrupted exposure
You cannot generate vitamin D if there's a glass
window between you and the sun. The UVB rays
needed for vitamin D production are absorbed by glass
and will not pass through to your skin.

3. Don't cover up with sunscreen
Even weak sunscreens will block the ability of your
skin to absorb the UVB rays and manufacture vitamin
D. However, once you have surpassed your 20-30
minutes of unprotected exposure, you should get out
of the sun or cover up with something. If you do
need sunscreen, find one that contains no chemicals.
Visit the *Environmental Working Group* website,
www.ewg.org, to find the safest products.

4. Protect your skin with food
Still worried that exposing your skin to sunlight is
harmful? Load up on anti-oxidant rich foods and
beneficial fats that will strengthen your skin cells and
help to protect them from sun damage. The way of

eating that I outlined in Part 2 of this book will have you covered, but in particular these foods include vegetables and fruits such as blueberries, raspberries, goji berries and pomegranates.

5. Have your Vitamin D levels tested regularly
The best way to find out whether you are deficient or not is to take yourself along to have a blood test. If you're aiming for optimal health, you will want your level to be in the 100–150 ng/ml range. The higher the better, for preventing and healing disease.

6. Take a supplement
During winter, or if you live in an area that gets minimal sun exposure, you may need to source a vitamin D3 supplement. The sun is the best way to obtain vitamin D but, when this isn't possible, you need to back yourself up. Be careful with supplementation though, because taking too large a dose can lead to vitamin D toxicity. This is why sunlight is the best source of vitamin D, as the body will only take and generate what it needs. If you think you need a supplement, check with your doctor or naturopath first. Then have your vitamin D levels checked regularly, to ensure you're not getting more than you need.

MOVEMENT

I have a confession to make. Up until recently, movement was one of the areas where I've failed to practise what I was preaching. I was doing yoga a few times a week, but I was never consistent. I allowed all sorts of excuses to justify the fact that I was a little bit lazy.

Back in my self-loathing phase, I'd promise myself that I would get up early and go for a run almost every morning. I even went as far as putting a note with 'Get out of bed, fatty!' next to my alarm clock, to try and coerce me out from out under the covers. It never worked. When I joined a gym, the temporary novelty encouraged me to go to classes and slog it out on the treadmill—until I got so over it that I found any excuse not to go, and ended up paying a monthly membership fee for something I never used.

It wasn't until I gave myself permission to stop exercising altogether that it subtly became a permanent part of my life. I quit the gym and accepted that I would never be an early morning runner, and opted for movement for the sake of mental balance over weight loss. It was then that I discovered Bikram yoga. I instantly fell in love. I loved how clean, balanced and strong it made me feel—both physically and mentally. It was no coincidence that I started up Bikram yoga around the same time that I began making changes to my diet and lifestyle. I was eating a super clean diet, my head was clear, and I naturally wanted to round out my transformation with exercise. However, if I had attempted Bikram back when I was a drug-popping, booze-addled, frozen meal-loving party girl, I doubt I would have fallen as madly in love with the practice as I did. Camel pose makes you want to puke enough as it is—imagine attempting it with a hangover!

Now, I move my ass on a daily basis. I wake up early every morning and climb up Mount Coolum (something I never thought I would be able to do). Then, in the afternoons, I might go to yoga, jump on my mini trampoline, or go for a run. You'll find that exercising first up in the morning makes the rest of your day flow better. You go through the day with peace of mind, knowing that movement has already been ticked off your to-do list.

You will **never** regret the decision to exercise. Just like with your diet, not all exercise activities suit everyone. You just have to try out a few and find the right one for you. Here are some suggestions:

- running, bouncing on a mini trampoline, swimming, team sports like touch football, boot camp, Cross Fit, classes at your local gym, cardio and weights at your local gym, dancing, hiking in the great outdoors, surfing, stand-up paddle boarding, boxing, tennis, Pilates, soft sand running, etc

Then there's yoga in all of its glorious forms:

- Vinyasa, Ashtanga, Power, Yin, Iyengar, Anusara, Bikram, Hatha, Jivamukti, Kundalini and many more

Making movement fun will transform it from being a chore and something you dread to a part of your routine that you love. Believe me when I tell you that this is possible! It all comes down to the **purpose** of your exercise. If the only reason you're exercising is to lose weight, it's going to be tricky to maintain. This is because your mind isn't in the present moment—you're future tripping to a time, place and body that doesn't exist, so you're going to hate the moment that you're currently living in. However, if you stay focused on the present moment and make being healthy and feeling amazing **in the present moment** the purpose of your exercise routine, it'll be much easier and enjoyable to stick to.

I use exercise as a form of meditation. I focus on my body and get out of my head. I feel my legs as I'm running, I focus on my breathing, and I mindfully take in the environment around me. When you exercise somewhere as beautiful as the beach, a park, or a mountain, it's easy to silence your mind by becoming so absorbed in the moment.

Need more inspiration to move? Here you go!

Exercise is one of the only ways to get your lymphatic system moving. Your lymphatic system doesn't have an in-built pump—exercise is the pump it needs to give it a kick start.

healthy lymph = healthy body

Exercise gets your heart pumping and boosts circulation. It will encourage freshly-oxygenated blood to be pumped around your body, flushing your cells with goodness. It's also the access key to your personal pharmacy of natural endorphins. In simple terms, exercise will improve your mood and make you happy!

Exercise clears your mind, enhances your mental capabilities, helps you lose weight, tones your body, leads to better and deeper sleep, and improves the health of your hormones to put the spark back in your sex life.

Exercise delivers oxygen to your lungs, helping you breathe more deeply, flooding your cells with freshly-oxygenated air, and alkalising your body. This all leads to the granddaddy of benefits: exercise prevents and helps to heal disease! If that doesn't inspire you to get up off your tushie and start moving, I don't know what will.

— SLEEP

If you're not getting enough sleep, or enough good quality sleep, you're not giving your body the chance it needs to cleanse and detoxify. Our bodies repair themselves when we're asleep. It's like when everyone leaves an office building for the night and the cleaners come in to do their thing. They need a good solid period of non-interruption to do their job effectively. The same goes for your body. Between the hours of 11pm and 4am, your body is cleansing, detoxifying and repairing. It's also producing melatonin, a hormone secreted by the pineal gland in the brain. Melatonin helps regulate other hormones and maintains the body's circadian rhythm; it slows down the ageing process; it strengthens the immune system; and it has strong antioxidant effects. The more melatonin your body has, the better you will feel.

I want to chat more about this circadian rhythm for just a moment. This is a natural internal clock that resets itself every 24 hours. Different chemicals are released in the body at times determined by this clock and depending on whether the clock thinks the body needs to be asleep or awake. This internal clock is set by light. Every time you turn on a light, you are resetting the rhythm and interrupting its work, so that the individual cells within the body don't release chemicals or produce the necessary proteins at the right time. So, when we stay up later than we should and wake up earlier than we should, we're forcing our bodies to work overtime and don't give them the chance they need to restore themselves. An out-of-whack circadian rhythm leads to an overworked body, which then leads to imbalances and fatigue, quickening the ageing process.

Tips for an awesome night's sleep

— Aim to be in bed by 9.30pm and asleep by 10pm.

— Create a nighttime ritual, to prepare your body for sleep. Just as it's important to not hit the ground running in the morning, it's just as important to wind down properly before going to bed.

— Dim the lights a couple of hours before you hit the hay. This will start the production of melatonin.

— Write in a journal before you go to bed, to get your thoughts out of your head.

— If you get up to go to the bathroom during the night, try to leave the light off or have as little light as possible. As soon as you turn on the light, you will cease all production of the important sleep aid melatonin. If you do need to have a light on in the bathroom, opt for a red/orange-coloured light, as this won't disrupt melatonin production as much. I keep a Himalayan salt lamp on in my bathroom, just in case I need to get up and pee during the night.

— If you still have trouble nodding off, I recommend getting your hands on a herb called valerian. You can buy it in capsule or tea form, and it has amazing calming powers. It's like a gentle sleeping pill that won't leave you feeling drowsy next day.

∞ AFFIRMATIONS

Generally, we have no trouble saying awful things to ourselves, predicting the worst, and letting irrational fears rule our thoughts. But when it comes to consistently thinking positively, we tend to struggle. The truth is that we have the power to choose our thoughts and, with a bit of practice, we can make a conscious effort to choose thoughts that will empower us, lift us up, and make us happy.

Repeating affirmations is a great way to dissolve limiting beliefs and reprogram our minds to think in our favour. When used often, affirmations create new pathways in our brains and teach us to think in a positive way. Keep them up for long enough and these positive thoughts will take the place of negative ones as our default thought patterns.

Because of their simplicity, affirmations are often disregarded or not taken as seriously as they deserve. But it's often these simple acts that create the most powerful changes. I use affirmations whenever I'm nervous about something, whenever I'm scared of something, or whenever I need to be talked down from some kind of emotional ledge. The most powerful one I've used is, *I love and accept myself.* As soon as I say that and keep it on repeat for a while, my subconscious mind picks up on the fact that I can do whatever it is I'm setting my mind to. Affirmations ground me and give me a reality check.

Choose a few of these affirmations to have on mental repeat. You'll be amazed at the simple, subtle shifts they create in your life.

family. You may find that some of the people around you are not very supportive. They might criticise you, ridicule you, try to undermine your choices, and act in a condescending and judgemental manner.

This happens a lot when we start eliminating certain foods from our diet, and those around us don't quite understand why we're doing it. If and when this happens, I want you to remember one thing: It's all them! It's all their stuff—not yours. Seeing you actually commit to making your life better will most likely cause them to look at their own lives. This can bring up any insecurities and discontentment that they are feeling, and will shine a light on the areas they know they want and need to change. If they're aware but aren't willing to make any changes just yet, it's possible that they're trying to cover up their self-loathing and insecurities by being all snarky towards you.

If and when this happens, just take a deep breath and take the compassionate road. If you feel it's right, calmly explain to them why you're doing what you're doing. And if they don't want a bar of it, just smile at them and send them love. This is when they need it most. We all get this stuff in our own time, and often just seeing you confidently leading by example will be all the inspiration they need.

Relationships that are fraught with drama are not worth it. When the people around you constantly trigger your stress response, it's time to be honest with yourself about whether these people need to be in your life—or to what extent they need to be in your life. Don't bring on lifestyle detriments just because you feel obliged to keep certain people in your life. From experience, I can say that when you let go of people who bring you down, you will attract people who will lift you up. But it's not until you make space for these new, amazing relationship assets that they will come your way.

∞ SPIRITUALITY

One of the best ways to diminish your cravings for the superficial trimmings of life is to cultivate a spiritual awareness and practice. I'm not saying you need to go to church, read the Bible, or even call yourself religious. This is different to that. Spirituality is simply about believing in a power greater than yourself, and understanding that there is something out there that is orchestrating this thing we call life—something that will always look after your back, no matter what.

Once you strengthen this belief, and hone in on this trust, it will allow you to see that you are never alone; you are always safe, and your life carries more meaning than you could ever imagine. When you believe that, fear is dissolved and you feel eternally supported. Suddenly even a packet of chocolate biscuits seems less alluring.

For me, spirituality is harnessed mostly through meditation, because this is when I'm connected to that place inside of me that I just know is a part of every other living thing on this planet. This is also the place that instantly reassures me that everything is always going to be okay. My definition of spirituality is trusting that we are always going to be taken care of.

Self-care

ꝏ Everything you do that has a positive impact on your body, mind and soul can be considered 'self-care'. Therefore, everything we've spoken about so far can, of course, be classified as just that. However, this chapter is dedicated to a few simple, cheap and quick practices that will really ramp up the love you show to your body.

ꝏ DRY BODY BRUSHING

Our skin is our largest organ, so it makes sense that we should pay it the same amount of respect that we do to our other organs. The easiest way to show your skin some loving is by taking to it with a dry body brush. Dry body brushing will boost circulation, stimulate your lymphatic system, sloth off dead skin, and open your pores.

This is a simple practice that can be done each morning, before you step into the shower. All you need to do is brush over your skin in long sweeping strokes, towards your heart. Start at your legs and work your way up. Pay particular attention to your thighs and buttocks to deal with cellulite;

brush over your armpits and groin area several times to stimulate your lymphatic nodes; and then move the brush around your stomach, starting by going down the left side to move your digestive system. Be careful when brushing over sensitive areas like your face and breasts.

Because dry body brushing calls for you to pay attention to your body, it's also a great way to bolster self-love. Repeat loving affirmations while you're brushing away.

⎯ OIL PULLING

I've found that, out of all of the weird and wacky detox processes I discuss on my website, oil pulling is the one that is most fascinating to people. I think this is because its list of benefits is so long, compared with how easy it is to do.

Oil pulling is simply this:

> Put a tablespoon of cold pressed organic oil in your mouth, swish it around for 20 minutes, and then spit it into the bin. Done. I use coconut oil because I love the way it tastes, and coconut oil has so many benefits. However, this practice is most traditionally done with sesame or sunflower oil.

Consistently doing this every day can lead to brighter and whiter teeth, healthier gums, clearer sinuses, clearer skin, better sleep, a clearer mind, no more bad breath, increased energy, alleviated allergies, regulated menstrual cycles, improved lymph system and improved PMS symptoms. All this, simply for swishing oil around your mouth. Pretty cool, right?

Oil pulling is an ancient Ayurvedic ritual, introduced to the modern world in 1992 by Dr F Karach MD. Dr Karach claimed that oil pulling could cure a variety of illnesses, ranging from heart disease and digestive troubles to hormonal disorders.

Bruce Fife, naturopathic physician and author of *Oil Pulling Therapy: Detoxifying and Healing the Body Through Oral Cleansing* says:

> *The oil acts like a cleanser. When you put it in your mouth and work it around your teeth and gums it 'pulls' out bacteria and other debris. As simple as it is, oil pulling has a very powerful detoxifying effect. Our mouths are home to billions of bacteria, viruses, fungi and other parasites and their toxins. Candida and streptococcus are common residents in our mouths. It's these types of germs and their toxic waste products that cause gum disease and tooth decay and contribute to many other health problems including arthritis and heart disease. Our immune system is constantly fighting these troublemakers. If our immune system becomes overloaded or burdened by excessive stress, poor diet, environmental toxins and such, these organisms can spread throughout the body causing secondary infections and chronic inflammation, leading to any number of health problems.*

Oil pulling is best done first thing in the morning on an empty stomach. I put the oil in my mouth and then jump back into bed to read or write in my journal. If I'm pressed for time, I'll swish while I'm showering. Never swallow the oil, as the swishing will render it full of toxins. Be sure to brush your teeth and rinse your mouth thoroughly afterwards. Sometimes I'll add a couple of drops of oregano oil to my coconut oil, to boost its antibacterial and antimicrobial properties.

The first few times I did this my gag reflexes reared themselves, and it was a little difficult keeping the oil in my mouth. But I persisted, and by the third day it was fine. If you have this problem too, I recommend sticking with it.

Some may disregard oil pulling because it is so simple (and we humans love to complicate everything). However it's so cheap, easy and backed up by so much anecdotal evidence that I couldn't ignore it. As a result, my teeth are whiter and my gums no longer bleed when I brush them.

— CLAY EATING

Yes, this is actually a thing! I promise I haven't gone over the edge. Thanks to the chemotherapy I had when I was first diagnosed with cancer, my body is still weighed down by heavy metals. Even without chemo poison, many of us are heavy metal contaminated; thanks to pollutants in the air, at the hairdresser, at the petrol station, in our seafood, in our water, in our cosmetics, in tattoos—and in pretty much everything else we consume. This is why I've taken to eating a spoonful of dirt each morning.

According to the book *The Clay Cure* by Ran Knishinsky, clay heals a wide range of illnesses including constipation, diarrhoea, anaemia, chronic infections, skin ailments such as eczema and acne, heavy metal poisoning, exposure to pesticides and other toxins, arthritis and stress. *Clay contains the minerals and energy that the defence mechanism needs; it improves bowel function and detoxifies the body of pollutants,* says John Tilden MD.

Clay particles carry a negative electrical charge, whereas impurities (or toxins) carry a positive electrical charge. When we eat clay, the positively-charged toxins are attracted by the negatively-charged edges of the clay mineral. An exchange reaction occurs, where the clay swaps its ions for those of the other substance. Electrically satisfied, it holds the toxin in suspension until the body can eliminate both. In layman's terms: we eat the clay, the clay binds to toxins, and then we poop both the toxins and the clay out.

People have been eating clay for yonks. In fact, over two hundred cultures worldwide eat dirt on a daily basis. In Europe, clay is sold for its gastrointestinal benefits and its purification properties. It's just that, for some reason, the idea of eating dirt disgusts most westerners—even though we are more than happy to consume pesticides, herbicides, chlorinated and fluoridated water, meats pumped with hormones and antibiotics, and other synthetic substances disguised as food. That's all the more reason why we should be eating clay, if you ask me! Even animals eat clay. They are instinctively drawn to clay and many herbivorous animals will eat clay after ingesting herbs loaded with tannins, a toxic substance.

The 'how to' of clay eating

It's actually more like drinking than eating. Each morning, I dissolve a teaspoon or two of edible earth in a cup of water, and then drink it down. I was a little wary at first, but the taste is totally inoffensive and it's very easy to drink. Look for either bentonite or montmorillonite. These are the most common and most sought after clays that are suitable for eating. Their ability to adsorb and absorb toxins is greater than that of clays in the other groups.

⁰⁰⁰⁰ NATURAL BEAUTY

If there's one piece of advice you take away from this section, let it be this:

> If you can't eat it or drink it,
> don't put it on your skin.

As I mentioned before, our skin is our largest organ, and everything that we apply to it is absorbed straight into our bloodstream. Whatever you put on your skin, hair, nails and teeth is absorbed straight into your body. However, applying chemicals to your skin can be even worse that ingesting them via the mouth because, when they're applied to the skin, we don't have the slight protection of them being filtered through the liver.

Commercial make-up, skin products and hair care products are full of toxic chemicals. They contain additives, preservatives and oils based on petrochemicals. None of these belong in the body. They accumulate and cause a heap of damage to your endocrine and immune systems, leading to weight gain, fertility issues, and pretty much all diseases. The good news is that there are plenty of organic, all-natural alternatives on the market. You just need to learn how to read labels and decipher ambiguous terms.

The thing with cosmetics is that no-one regulates the safety of their ingredients. Cosmetics companies can basically add whatever they want to their products, and no-one will

In other natural home-related news, open your windows to let natural light and air filter your home; display plants around the place to mop up impurities in the air; and keep your home clean and clutter-free. All of this will not only do wonders for your mental state, but it will greatly affect the health of your body. Houseguests will always leave thinking, *Man, I wish my place was that Zen!*

THE MINDSET BEHIND PERMANENT TRANSFORMATION

CHAPTER TWELVE

∞∞ Let's be honest; it's not lack of information that causes us to make poor choices for ourselves. Like when it's a Friday night and we sit on the couch devouring an entire tub of ice cream ... you don't need to be a nutritionist to know that's not a good idea! Or like the time when I drank so much wine that I thought it was a brilliant idea to steal the microphone from the band at the club I was at, and was then asked to leave the venue. And then, when I had nothing to do besides wait out the front for my friends, I didn't honestly think that eating an entire hot box full of something the vendor described as 'mystery meat' was a healthy choice for me.

No, it's not lack of knowledge that causes us to do these things (you've done them too, right?). Something else is happening in our brains, and it has everything to do with the five elements I'm going to unpack in this chapter. Bad decisions may make for good stories, but they don't make for sustainable health and happiness. If you really want to create lasting healthy habits and a permanent lifestyle transformation, it's important to understand the mindset that is needed before this can happen.

∞ MINDSET SECRET #1 ⦚ SELF-LOVE

I want to let you in on a little secret: willpower doesn't actually exist. We do things out of self-love or self-loathing—nothing else. And it's self-love that is the foundation that makes healthy habits stick.

Louise Hay says that most, if not all, of our problems stem from the personal belief that we are not good enough. When you think about it, all that judging and berating we do to ourselves has to show up somewhere. And it does so in our ability to make positive choices for ourselves.

Without self-love, we're constantly trying to fill a void that cannot be filled. We look for external gratification and superficial fulfilment, in the hope that it will make us happy. When someone is seriously lacking in self-love, they will attempt to make up for it with food, alcohol, drugs, sex, shopping, or some other external temporary band-aid. But, of course, none of this works and we just end up in a vicious self-loathing cycle. We constantly look outside ourselves for the answer; but this will never work, because happiness can only truly be sought when we're willing to go within.

Then there are the wars we wage against our own bodies. When we treat our bodies like they're our worst enemies, how can we expect them to love us back with good health, vibrancy and energy? When we go on a diet, it's like we're declaring war against our bodies. We 'battle the bulge' and 'fight the fat' and approach weight loss from a place of anger and hate. We hate how we look, we hate our lack of willpower, and we hate the fact that, no matter how much we try to deprive ourselves of tasty food, the diet never works. Not in the long run, anyway. This is because we're going about it completely the wrong way.

Fighting against what is doesn't solve anything, because it doesn't deal with the reasons why things are the way they are. Everything in our lives is there for a particular reason, and for something to exist it means that we've created an environment for it to be a possibility. If disease exists in the body, it means we've created an internal environment that allows that to happen. If weight is an issue, it means that something is going on beneath the surface that has caused weight to be an issue. Weight gain and disease are simply symptoms of a deeper imbalance.

You can't wage a war against yourself and expect to win. Even if it's a war fought with green juice and kale! To achieve what it is that you're truly pursuing, which I'm guessing is peace, health and happiness, you need to be ready to wave the white flag in front of whatever it is that you're fighting against and be willing to get to the core of the issue. You need to first accept what is for what it is—no matter how much you've branded it as a negative part of your life—and then get busy with the practice of authentic, deep self-love. If your intention is founded on self-hatred, fear or some other devious motive, all of the green veggies in the world won't help. But when you lay down a solid foundation of self-love, anything you build on top of it will stay in place for good.

My greatest shift came when I was told that I had to stop doing things out of fear of dying, and start doing them out of an unshakeable love for myself. That piece of wisdom rocked me to my core. From that moment I stopped drinking juices, meditating and putting coffee up my backside because I thought I 'should' do these things so that I wouldn't die. I started doing them—and doing them with passion—because I loved myself so much that I wanted to live. When fear is the prime motivator, results will be shallow and fickle. Love is the only motivation that will allow you to create a truly happy and healthy life.

How to cultivate self-love

1. Stop wishing for things to be different

When I was a teen, I was forever wishing that I had bigger boobs and smaller thighs. I would have traded my soul for these things; I thought they were so crucial to my success in the world. These days I'm absolutely content with my petite chest and rounded booty. But there's still something I work on every day concerning acceptance of myself: my left hand and arm. As a result of the chemo I had, my left hand and arm are pretty damaged. They have next to no strength and my left middle finger is fused at the knuckle and curled over into my palm. It's incredibly frustrating when it comes time to do flat-palmed postures in yoga, or when opening jars. I can also become self-conscious about the way it looks. My left arm is covered in scars, it's swollen, and those who don't know my story stare at it when I'm out and about. It's still very easy for me to slip on my pity party hat and call in the violins.

I have to remind myself on a daily basis that there's absolutely no point in wallowing in self-pity and wishing for things to be different. Wishing for things to be different is pointless. More than that, it's counter-productive. While we're busy wishing for things to be different, we're missing the point of why things are the way they are. There's magic in our circumstances. Everything in our lives is there for a particular reason. Surrendering to the reasons and responding to the messages and calls is not only our job; it makes life a heck of a lot more enjoyable. Practising acceptance of everything in your life—from the way you look to the diseases through which your body speaks to you—is the first step in cultivating authentic self-love. Complete acceptance is having your own back, no matter what.

Acceptance is something you can practise, even when you slip up and fall back into old habits. Don't beat yourself up and berate yourself. Don't judge yourself. Don't let yourself become ravaged by guilt. Simply recognise that you haven't made the best choice, and then gently remind yourself that you always have the power to choose something different. The thing is, we have an opportunity to make a positive choice every single moment of every single day. So, if you slip up, use the next moment to make a better choice. Guilt and self-sabotage will always do more damage than indulgence.

2. Practise gratitude

Paying homage to your blessings is like stepping onto the self-love fast track. What could be more loving that showing gratitude for everything that you have in your life—both the blessings and the lessons? Nothing, that's what. Gratitude is also our most powerful tool when it comes to cultivating happiness. It's almost impossible to be unhappy when you're sitting in a place of gratitude. The universe rewards grateful people so, when you show gratitude for what you already have, you will always receive more to be grateful for. It's a no-brainer, really.

I recommend two methods for practising gratitude on a daily basis:

- Keep a gratitude journal

  Either every morning when you wake up or every evening before you go to bed, take inventory of everything you have to be grateful for in your life, by making a list in your journal. These can be things as large as the people you're lucky enough to have love you, to as small as the nourishing food you have stocked in your fridge. It's also good to write about the challenges you're experiencing, and to attribute the lessons as blessings. Your list may look pretty much the same each day, so try your best to add a few different things as well. You'll be surprised by just how much goodness you have to be thankful for.

- Say 'thank you' through the day

I like to pause at random times throughout the day and just whisper a little 'thank you' to no-one in particular. I look for things like the vibrancy of a gorgeous green tree, the blue hue in the sky or a yummy salad or smoothie I've made for myself. Get into the habit of showing gratitude for little things, and you'll find you're able to be happy for no reason at all.

3. **Alone time**

Quality alone time is the foundation for a healthy relationship with yourself. Alone time allows you to get to know yourself better, get a real understanding of who are as a person, discover your authentic self, and then fall in love with it. You can't avoid yourself when you are the only one there to claim your attention. When you regularly spend time by yourself, you start to consider yourself as your own best friend. You cherish and honour the relationship you have with yourself. I'm nowhere near my best self unless I have sufficient time by myself. This is the reason why I love doing enemas so much (perfect excuse to lock myself in the bathroom with a good book for 30 minutes) and why my favourite thing to do is hop into bed with a cup of tea and a healthy dessert, to watch something trashy on the telly.

Even though I'm an only child, and so had to master the art of solo entertainment at a pretty young age, it wasn't until my early adult years that I was content to hang out by myself. I always thought I needed other people around me to validate my worth, or I thought that I was missing out on something if I was at home by myself. I'm an introvert by nature, and these days I'm happy to admit that. I'm also happy to admit that I crave alone time just as much (or if not more) as I crave love and attention from my love. To me, time alone is as essential as breathing.

4. **Repeat this affirmation: I love and accept myself**
Out of all of the affirmations you can say, this is the one that's going to help form and cement that special bond you want to have with yourself. The more you can have this mantra on repeat in your mind, the more effective it will be. It will seem silly at first; but I promise you that, if you stick with it, powerful shifts will begin to occur. I repeat this affirmation as soon as I wake up in the morning, when I start and end my meditation practice, when I'm in the shower, when I'm driving, and at any other time that I need to remind myself that I'm on my own team. If I'm feeling nervous about something, or fear starts to creep into my mind, I console myself with this mantra. It reminds me that, no matter what, I love and accept myself.

5. **Mirror work**
When was the last time you looked at yourself in the mirror, looked directly into your own eyes and said, 'I love you [insert your name here]'. Most of us look in the mirror and search for flaws. For the next 21 days, I want you to say, 'I love you [insert your name here]' every time you look at yourself in the mirror.

Look intently into your own eyes and tell yourself how freaking amazing you are.

If you're in the privacy of your own home, say it out loud. If not, just say it in your head. At first it might feel a little awkward and funny. However I promise that, after a while, it will become much easier. By the end of 21 days, saying 'I love you' every time you catch your reflection will be a natural reaction. You won't be able to pass by a store window without showering your awesome self in praise.

Once this step becomes a habit, you'll notice some amazing shifts starting to take place. You'll soften and be more compassionate—not just to yourself, but also to everyone around you. You'll readily forgive yourself, and you'll find that you don't criticise yourself as much. You'll gain confidence and stand up for yourself. You'll see that you are so much more than your body. You'll connect with yourself on a spiritual level, and see the perfection and innocence in your true self.

It's important to combine your words with an equally self-loving feeling. Don't just say 'I love you' while in your mind you're really thinking: 'You're a big fat mess'. If you don't feel the words, it's pointless.

If you have trouble saying, 'I love you' to yourself, ask yourself what you're so scared of. You might find it confronting, but I urge you to just go with it. Keep connecting with the feeling of love, and don't listen to the voice in your head that tells you that you've got fat thighs or too many chins. Feel love running through your body; let it plump up your cells and swell your heart. Say 'I wholeheartedly, unconditionally love you no matter what.'

No matter what you look like, complete acceptance is the most powerful place to start. Keep doing this—even when the critical voice pipes up—and soon you will wholeheartedly believe it. It just takes commitment and willingness to go there. Don't listen to the voice in your head; just sink into the feeling. It's a slow, gradual process to feel what that feels like. Self-love is a daily, moment-to-moment practice.

6. **Be gentle and kind with yourself**
Treat yourself the way a loving mother would treat her child. Practise self-forgiveness, self-compassion, self-acceptance and patience. Don't take yourself too seriously. Let go of perfectionist tendencies and release your need to control situations. When you mess up, be the first to console yourself and tell yourself that you deeply love and accept yourself anyway. When things don't go your way, remind yourself that it's probably because something better is on its way. Be on your own side and always, always, always have your own back.

— MINDSET SECRET #2 ⦙ STOP ALL OF THE COMPARING

Back when my mind was easily won over by self-loathing thoughts, it was generally images in magazines or on telly that did the tormenting. I was a magazine junkie, consuming every new title to hit news stands. Working in magazines didn't help either. For the most part, the girls who work on the glossy pages really are every bit as polished and stylish as the girls gracing the pages. Walking through the halls of 'magazine land' every day left me with a serious case of comparison-itis.

These days we have so many more aesthetics to compare ourselves with. There's *Facebook, Twitter, Instagram, Pinterest,* and a gazillion blogs. Thanks to all of the self-love practising I do, I'm nowhere near as ravaged by the self-judgement and all of the 'I wish I looked like that' thinking that would usually set in after seeing a stream of gorgeous bodies. Heck, I can even settle in with my boyfriend and watch the *Victoria's Secret* show and join him in admiring the girls. Once upon a time, this would have had me hating myself for days afterwards. Instead of comparing, I'm inspired. I use my *Instagram* feed to inspire me to take care of myself with a clean diet and exercise.

Send genuine kudos to those you're envious of. They'll feel it, and it will prevent you from falling victim to jealousy. When you compare yourself to other people, it's like instantly telling yourself that you're not good enough. It's the number one thing we all need to stop doing if we're going to have a chance at cultivating self-love. Comparison instantly robs you of any positive feelings you have towards yourself. Nothing good comes of it. The reality is that, any time you judge someone for something that they have and that you want, you will automatically block that something from coming your way. So, whenever you see someone who you're a little envious of, celebrate it. Be genuinely happy for them. Send those feelings of jealousy back to where they came from, and let your ego know that there's no place for such blessing-blocking thoughts in your world.

Another thing. We can only recognise in others that which we have within ourselves. Therefore, if you're jealous of something that someone else has achieved or a particular personality trait that you find endearing, this means that you have the ability to bring this forward from within yourself. Switch comparison and jealousy for fiery inspiration.

∞ MINDSET SECRET #3 ⁞ YOU DON'T HAVE TO GIVE ANYTHING UP

My brilliant friend, comedian Kyle Cease, once said that we humans have a lot of trouble letting go of things that are no longer serving us, because we can't see what we are going to gain in their place. This is true for every area our lives: careers, relationships and food.

I absolutely resented having to leave my job at *Dolly* magazine, because I didn't think I would be able to land a gig that sweet again. It took me ages to break up with my ex-boyfriend, even though I knew he wasn't the one for me, because my mind was telling me that I wouldn't be able to find someone who loved me like that again. And then, when it was evident that saving my life would require a complete diet overhaul, I absolutely hated that I had to give up eating Thai takeaway, pizza and meat pies. How does one live without Thai food, I wondered? How does one make it through Friday without fried chicken Friday? I'd always had trouble saying 'no' to fries with my meals, let alone giving up the meal altogether.

I thought my life was over, and this was because I couldn't see what I would gain as replacements to my old preservative-laden favourite foods. I had no idea about things like cacao, natural sweeteners and coconut oil. I had absolutely no idea that I would be able to recreate healthy versions of these favourite foods and that, by doing so, I would be able to eat them as much as I wanted, without the old familiar guilt trip creeping in.

One of the reasons why diets don't work is because they're all about deprivation. They take your favourite foods away from you and provide poor substitutes in their place. Who's going to get excited about sitting on the couch on a Friday night with a powdered shake or a couple of dry rice cakes? Or worse, they are replaced with 'fat free' treats that trick you into thinking you're eating something yummy and guilt-free, only to leave you feeling unsatisfied and wanting more, because your body hasn't recognised the processed crap as food. Dieting actually makes you fatter. When we tell ourselves that we have to give up something that we love, our minds instantly go into resistance mode and we end up rebelling, by eating more chocolate cake. It's pure sorcery, I tell you.

Once you fully understand that removing something from your life only makes room for something better to take its place, change and transformation will be a much smoother process.

~ MINDSET SECRET #4 ⦙ LOOK AT WHAT'S NOT WORKING IN YOUR LIFE, THEN DO THE OPPOSITE

In so many ways, I'm incredibly lucky that I was diagnosed with cancer at such a young age. It was my body's way of telling me that what I was doing was no longer serving me. It was the wake-up call I needed, to start doing the direct opposite of what I was doing. These days, I am in bed by 10pm every night; I get high on green juice; and I haven't had a hangover since November 2009.

Our bodies speak to us in whispers, so tune in and listen to what yours is telling you. Take an honest look at your life. Be truthful with yourself. If something is no longer working, and you know what that is, do the exact opposite.

If you aren't getting enough sleep—sleep more. If you're overwhelmed—simplify your life. If you don't eat enough vegetables—drink veggie juices and eat salad. If you're constantly eating on the run or don't have time to prepare meals—seriously, assess that now and make the time. Just make the time! We all have the same amount of hours in the day. If you don't exercise enough, then find a form you enjoy and do it. Stop making excuses. Stop making plans to make changes. All you need to do is look at what's no longer serving you, eliminate it and replace it with something that will. It's that simple.

Stop telling yourself that everything is all right in moderation. Why would you want to live a moderately brilliant life, when you can live to your absolute potential and reap the benefits of such a commitment? Why would you want to cheat yourself out of anything less than you deserve and that you are capable of?

— MINDSET SECRET #5 ⦙ BE IN THE PRESENT MOMENT

I touched on this a little back, when we were talking about exercise. But a topic this powerful deserves a section all of its own. Actually, it deserves a book of its own but Eckhart Tolle has already got that covered (*The Power Of Now*—read it ASAP).

One of the ways our minds sabotage us and keep us from making healthy changes is by pulling us away from the present moment to a place where we project made-up fears onto our current situation. So, one of the biggest secrets for transforming your life is learning how to be present.

Our egos live in the past or the future. So, when we keep our minds focused on the present moment, it's impossible for our egos to start whispering in our ears. Past dwelling and future tripping are breeding grounds for health-sabotaging spawn like fear, anxiety and worry—emotions that lead us to crave comfort foods. When we skip ahead and live in the future, we generally think things will be worse than what they are. I'm speaking mostly about healthy changes when I say that. Think about the last time you thought about making changes that you know you need to make. It may have been giving up certain foods, starting an exercise routine or practising meditation. When these things are foreign to us—when we're starting from a place where we're yet to give them a try—we generally perceive them as much harder and more difficult to maintain than they actually are.

When we want to start eating foods that are healthy, our minds will take us into the future and tell us that it won't be enjoyable there. So we give up, and go back to foods that are familiar. If you were to sit down and mindfully eat a gorgeous packed salad, you would be focused on how amazing the subtle flavours in the plants are. But if you were to eat the salad, while at the same time thinking about a meat pie you ate a while ago or dreaming about eating pizza, you would hate every bite of that salad.

The same goes for meditation. When we stay present, concentrating on our breathing and feeling the sensations in our body, it's quite easy and enjoyable to sit still for a length of time. However, when our minds fool us into thinking about how long we have to sit still for, we instantly think we're bored and we become inclined to get up and busy ourselves with tasks.

Touching on the exercise thing again, if we were to climb a mountain by continuously looking at how far we have to go, we would be tempted to give up. However, if we just stayed focused on the present moment, we would be content. We would be able to just do whatever task we're doing—we wouldn't be tripping out over how hard the task is, or how bored we are—we would simply be doing whatever it is we set out to do. When we stay grounded in the now, there's no room for the sabotaging thoughts that are certain to set in, when we think about the past or project into the future.

Being present seems like a simple concept, and it should be. However, we're so conditioned to be anything besides present that it's one of the toughest things we can master. We love a good distraction, especially when our circumstances are a tad uncomfortable. Keeping our attention on the now is a moment-by-moment, breath-by-breath challenge that we will only begin to grasp when we commit to a consistent practice. Even those who have been at it for a while need to keep it up with constant acts of anchoring. It's just like strengthening muscles at the gym. You may reach a point where you're happy with how you look but, if you halt your exercises, you'll quickly return back to a softer form. The same applies for training for your mind to stay present. I have a four-step process I use, whenever I feel my mind starting to wig out, by dragging me away from the moment at hand. It goes like this:

- Focus on your breath by listening and feeling deep inhales and long, slow exhales.

- Drop out of your head and into your body, by consciously feeling sensations in your body. Feel your feet firmly planted on the ground, and then attempt to feel your body from the inside out.

- Listen to the sounds around you and let your ears search for the subtle sounds in the background. Then listen to the silence between the sounds.

- Meditatively look around, slowing taking in objects that are around you, without labelling them.

If this doesn't work, I know it's time for more drastic measures. I'll either step outside to be among nature, go for a walk on the beach, or head for my meditation stool for a quick session of stillness. When my head's clear again, it's much easier to stay rooted in the moment.

EXPERT WORD ¦ DEEPAK CHOPRA

The most important time in your life is right now.

The most important person is the one that is in front of you right now.

The most important activity is the one you are doing right now.

Deepak Chopra is an American physician, a holistic health guru, and one of the world's most notable alternative medicine practitioners.

ENDING THE WAR

CHAPTER THIRTEEN

∞ When I was in high school, I incessantly wished to wake up one morning and magically transform into one of those people who could eat whatever they wanted, and never put on weight. You know, one of those people blessed with a 'fast metabolism'. I had friends like that and I envied them something fierce. I had a major case of comparison-itis, and this same brush painted every area of my life. Everything was just so hard. I ate with my growing bum and thighs always in the back of my mind. I exercised with an image of a stick figure in my mind. I shopped for clothes with a dark cloud of self-hatred looming over me as I looked over at my girlfriends purchasing clothes I loved, only in sizes I couldn't fit into. I experienced all of this angst, and I've never in my life been overweight.

This was all just a tortured result of deep conditioning, of growing up in a backward world that doesn't teach us things like eating for nourishment, exercising for wellbeing and falling in love with every inch of ourselves. I also hated myself for being partial to foods like creamy pasta, bread and hot chips, and I wished that the rule in life would be that tasty food could also be healthy.

It turns out that my wish came true; but the catalyst wasn't a magic wand, it was simply a re-education and a complete transformation of my relationship with food. It all started with my world falling apart.

In hindsight, this needed to happen, so that my previously-held beliefs could be shaken up and I could rebuild my body and mind from scratch. Without the cancer diagnosis, I don't think my mind would have been cracked open wide enough to consider the idea that everything I'd been taught about food, nourishment and self-confidence was fabricated by the misinformed. I was stubborn, a little arrogant, and had a tendency to roll my eyes at new ideas that I wasn't comfortable considering. If I were around someone who chose salad over pizza, I would judge them. If someone started cutting things from their diet like wheat, dairy or sugar, I would be very quick to think of them as a pain in the butt and a little crazy. And if someone were to go as far as cut meat from their diet, I thought they were just going through a phase. No-one can swear off bacon forever, I thought. When I became the one who was pedantic about my food choices, abstaining from anything that would taint the pure temple that is my body, no-one was more surprised at myself than me.

For me, the beginning of this journey felt like I'd fallen down the rabbit hole in *Alice in Wonderland*. I was given good reason to question absolutely everything about the world I'd been living in—the food, the people, the rules, and the commonly-held beliefs. As I did this, I could see I was rocking the boat. My blog, which I was using to air all of the information I was learning, received so much praise. But I also attracted my fair share of criticism from people who felt uneasy about the idea that everything we'd been taught about food and health may well be a lie. My friendships also changed. As I became more interested in enhancing my life with green juice and quinoa, rather than chemicals and cocktails, I realised I was no longer like anyone I had around me. The tight friendships I'd had since I was a teenager have remained in my life, but they began to loosen. The more steps I took along this new path, the louder the creak I left on the step I was leaving.

Thankfully, I didn't let these uncomfortable shifts and often unpleasant situations deter me from the road that I knew deep down would lead me to the greatest blessings. The whole time I was making changes and passionately transforming my life, I had this strong intuition guiding me. And then, before I knew it, I was on the other side of the struggle, looking back with complete understanding of why everything happened the way that it did. The cancer, the criticism, the changes: all of this had to happen for me to have another shot at living out this life to my absolute full potential, as the best version and highest expression of me.

I'm writing this final chapter with so much gratitude overflowing from my heart. Thanks to my body, its brilliant wake-up call and subsequent lifestyle changes, I now live every single moment with pure intention. I wake up every morning so excited to be awarded the privilege of living my life and living it in a body that is so damn gorgeous, clever, and all-round amazing. I've attracted the kinds of friendships that are so supportive, nurturing and nourishing. My relationship with my partner is more caring, respectful and more fun than I knew was possible. My career is out-of-this-world amazing, something I would happily do for free, and something that I'm endlessly grateful for.

Cancer is my greatest teacher, and I can honestly say that it was the biggest blessing the universe could have given me. It clearly knew that I wouldn't have listened to any other logic, when it came to persuading me to change my ways. Thanks to the wisdom and lessons from the past few years, I'm now a better friend (to myself and others), a better girlfriend, a better daughter, a better pug mother, and a better person all round. Every single part of my life is better, because of my pledge to live in alignment with what my body needs and wants. It was all more than worth it.

Even though this is the path that was necessary for me, and I wouldn't change one bit of it, I also wouldn't wish cancer upon anyone. I truly hope that you're open to taking direction from your body, before it resorts to yelling at you with a terminal diagnosis. Prevention is where it's at, my friend, and I want you to promise yourself that you'll take it seriously. The lifestyle advice we've chewed over in these pages is first and foremost about delivering your body the most vibrant, optimum, incredible health ever. Weight loss, shiny hair, clear skin and endless energy are amazing by-products.

That's the message I want to leave you with. Whenever you begin to question your ability to transform your life, or your motivation begins to wane, I want you to conjure up a vision of the life you know you deserve to be living.

If you're here, holding this book in your hands and reading these words, you deserve to be living the absolute best life you can possibly imagine. This is the birthright of every single one of us. The only thing that is holding this dream back from manifestation is the uninspired choices we make. But remember, the good news is that we have the power to make a different choice every single moment.

It's time to end the war—with ourselves, with each other, and with the laws of nature and the universe. It's time to end the war with food. Food—real food—deserves to be prioritised above anything else, and cherished for the life-giving rocket fuel that it is. It's time to stop fighting, to stop betraying ourselves, to listen to what our bodies are trying to tell us, to accept that things are the way they are for a reason, and to step into our own unique potential to create the kinds of lives we are supposed to be living. It's time to recognise what an incredible gift it is to reside in bodies that are so intelligent and resilient, and it's time to stop abusing this gift. It's time to honestly look at our lives and take ownership of every element of them.

But instead of blaming ourselves for the way we look, feel and live, it's time to recognise that, if we had the power to create what we have, we also have the power to create something different. Something better. Something that reflects how amazing we are when we strip away all of our crappy conditioning and limiting beliefs. It's time to break free of the shackles of common default excuses like, 'I don't have the time to be healthy' or 'I can't afford to be healthy' and radically take control of how our lives look and feel. Every single person on this planet has the power to choose differently in support of their health and happiness—even if that choice is as simple as thinking differently and letting the changes flow from there. Once you change your thinking, nothing else will stay the same.

It's also time to free ourselves from the shackles of perfection, and the belief that if we're not 100 per cent perfect 100 per cent of the time, weight, wrinkles and illness will set in. Do your absolute best, but also be gentle with yourself. The benefit of a healthy regime can be measured by how your mind copes when you stray from it slightly. If you tear into yourself, it's time to come back to self-love and self-compassion and remind yourself that it's the actions you take daily—not every now and then—that have the most profound affect on your health and life. Always act from love, not fear.

I want you to do a quick visualisation exercise with me:

Close your eyes and imagine yourself in the future as your ideal self; with your body strong, and your mind clear and focused. Picture what you look like, what you are doing, who you are surrounded by and—most importantly—how you are feeling. Think about how you feel about your body, how you feel about your relationships, how you feel about your career, and how you feel about yourself overall. Be as vividly detailed as you possibly can.

Now, get the you that is in the room right now to walk up to that ideal you and, as you look at the end result of your transformation, let the ideal you tell current you what an easy and enjoyable ride it has been, and how amazing the transformational journey has been. Have future you tell current you that everything you could ever imagine for yourself is more than possible, as long as you stay loyal to your dreams. Have future you then tell current you that it was all definitely worth it. Then, give future you a big hug before opening your eyes.

Do this visualisation exercise every day, and allow it to give you the fuel you need to keep making choices in favour of your dreams. It's inevitable that the road to transformation is going to be a bit bumpy. The only thing you have to worry about is being radically kind to yourself at all times and using this as the lens through which to live your life.

It's time to end the war. No more deprivation, no more dieting, no more guilt, no more torture and no more struggle. It's time to relish the fact that we can have our cake and eat it too, and that the universe is a friendly place that is here to support us, as long as we're willing to support ourselves. We don't have to choose between having fun and being healthy. The food that we love can love us back. And, above all else, when we truly make peace with ourselves, peace will ricochet out into every other area of our lives and mirror back to us a world in which everything feels right.

Peace out
Jess x

To Yvette Luciano. I can't even begin to describe how much your support, vision and nothing-is-impossible attitude means to me.

To my agency, Harry M Miller Group and my agent Lee Sutherland. Another family I'm privileged to be part of.

To my soul sisters: Melissa Ambrosini, Rachel MacDonald, Tara Bliss, Susana Frioni, Nicola Chatham, Amanda Rootsey and Yvette Luciano (again). Thank you for helping me create the wave, for being an endless source of inspiration, for being the perfect mix of crazy fun, woo-woo and fierce ambition, and for being the best group of friends I could ever ask for. You guys blow my mind.

To my best friend and soul mate, Melanie Elliott. You were the first person to ever suggest that I look into this weird world called "natural medicine". Thank you for 17 years of the kind of friendship that movies are made of.

To my love Tallon. Thank you for being so patient and supportive, for being my personal chef, my style consultant, my best friend, and for making life so much fun. You're my favourite person in the world.

To my fur baby Edie for being my constant, grunting, squish-faced companion.

And, saving the biggest acknowledgements for last, an eternal thank you goes out to my parents. I could fill another book with gratitude for everything you guys have done for me. Everything I do, am and have I owe to you. Best parents ever!

RESOURCES

Come and hang with me in these corners of the web ...

My website:
http://www.thewellnesswarrior.com.au/

My coaching program:
http://lifestyletransformationguide.com/

Facebook:
https://www.facebook.com/thewellnesswarrior

Instagram:
http://instagram.com/jessainscough

Twitter:
https://twitter.com/JessAinscough

NOTES

We hope you enjoyed this Hay House book. If you'd like to receive our online catalogue featuring additional information on Hay House books and products, or if you'd like to find out more about the Hay Foundation, please contact:

Hay House Australia Pty. Ltd.,
18/36 Ralph St., Alexandria NSW 2015
Phone: +61 2 9669 4299 • *Fax:* +61 2 9669 4144
www.hayhouse.com.au

Published and distributed in the USA by:
Hay House, Inc., P.O. Box 5100, Carlsbad, CA 92018-5100
Phone: (760) 431-7695 • *Fax:* (760) 431-6948
www.hayhouse.com®

Published and distributed in the United Kingdom by:
Hay House UK, Ltd., Astley House, 33 Notting Hill Gate,
London, W11 3JQ • *Phone:* 44-203-675-2450 • *Fax:* 44-203-675-2451
www.hayhouse.co.uk

Published and distributed in the Republic of South Africa by:
Hay House SA (Pty), Ltd., P.O. Box 990, Witkoppen 2068
Phone/Fax: 27-11-467-8904
www.hayhouse.co.za

Published in India by:
Hay House Publishers India, Muskaan Complex, Plot No. 3, B-2,
Vasant Kunj, New Delhi 110 070
Phone: 91-11-4176-1620 • *Fax:* 91-11-4176-1630
www.hayhouse.co.in

Distributed in Canada by:
Raincoast Books, 2440 Viking Way, Richmond, B.C. V6V 1N2
Phone: 1-800-663-5714 • *Fax:* 1-800-565-3770
www.raincoast.com

Take Your Soul on a Vacation
Visit **www.HealYourLife.com®** to regroup, recharge, and reconnect with
your own magnificence. Featuring blogs, mind-body-spirit news, and
life-changing wisdom from Louise Hay and friends.

Visit **www.HealYourLife.com®** today!